Living with Hearing Loss

Don McFerran is a consultant ear, nose and throat surgeon, working in Colchester, the UK's oldest town. He studied Natural Sciences at Queens' College Cambridge and then Clinical Medicine at Addenbrooke's Hospital, Cambridge. He has a particular interest in hearing loss and tinnitus. He has written numerous scientific papers and book chapters and has co-authored two books, including the sister volume to this book, *Living with Tinnitus and Hyperacusis* (Sheldon Press, 2010). He has a long relationship with the British Tinnitus Association (BTA), first as a member of its Professional Advisers Committee and more recently as a Trustee of the charity.

Lucy Handscomb trained as a hearing therapist 20 years ago and has worked in several audiology clinics offering counselling, advice and communication training to adults of all ages as they learn to adjust to hearing loss. She now teaches audiology students at University College, London, specializing in psychosocial aspects of hearing loss and rehabilitation skills. She runs regular short courses and has written several articles and book chapters on audiological rehabilitation. She is currently working towards her PhD at the University of Nottingham, which focuses on psychological reactions to tinnitus.

Cherilee Rutherford is the course director for the MSc Advanced Audiology programme at the UCL Ear Institute in London and lecturer in Amplification and Aural Rehabilitation to students in audiology. Her educational background is in speech–language therapy and audiology and she obtained a master's degree in health science and a clinical doctorate in audiology from Nova Southeastern University, Florida. Cherilee has worked clinically in both private practice and public health sectors, and also has experience working in the hearing instrument manufacturing industry before joining the academic world. Her research interests include music and amplification, tinnitus, and the impact of foreign accents on speech understanding in the hearing impaired population.

Overcoming Common Problems Series

Selected titles

A full list of titles is available from Sheldon Press,
36 Causton Street, London SW1P 4ST and on our website at
www.sheldonpress.co.uk

Breast Cancer: Your treatment choices
Dr Terry Priestman

Chronic Fatigue Syndrome: What you need to know
Dr Megan A. Arroll

Cider Vinegar
Margaret Hills

Coping Successfully with Chronic Illness: Your healing plan
Neville Shone

Coping Successfully with Shyness
Margaret Oakes, Professor Robert Bor and Dr Carina Eriksen

Coping with Difficult Families
Dr Jane McGregor and Tim McGregor

Coping with Epilepsy
Dr Pamela Crawford and Fiona Marshall

Coping with Guilt
Dr Windy Dryden

Coping with Liver Disease
Mark Greener

Coping with Memory Problems
Dr Sallie Baxendale

Coping with Obsessive Compulsive Disorder
Professor Kevin Gournay, Rachel Piper and Professor Paul Rogers

Coping with Schizophrenia
Professor Kevin Gournay and Debbie Robson

Coping with Thyroid Disease
Mark Greener

Depressive Illness: The curse of the strong
Dr Tim Cantopher

The Diabetes Healing Diet
Mark Greener and Christine Craggs-Hinton

The Empathy Trap: Understanding antisocial personalities
Dr Jane McGregor and Tim McGregor

Epilepsy: Complementary and alternative treatments
Dr Sallie Baxendale

Fibromyalgia: Your treatment guide
Christine Craggs-Hinton

Hay Fever: How to beat it
Dr Paul Carson

The Heart Attack Survival Guide
Mark Greener

Helping Elderly Relatives
Jill Eckersley

The Holistic Health Handbook
Mark Greener

How to Eat Well When You Have Cancer
Jane Freeman

How to Stop Worrying
Dr Frank Tallis

The Irritable Bowel Diet Book
Rosemary Nicol

Living with Complicated Grief
Professor Craig A. White

Living with IBS
Nuno Ferreira and David T. Gillanders

Making Sense of Trauma: How to tell your story
Dr Nigel C. Hunt and Dr Sue McHale

Overcoming Fear: With mindfulness
Deborah Ward

Overcoming Loneliness
Alice Muir

Overcoming Stress
Professor Robert Bor, Dr Carina Eriksen and Dr Sara Chaudry

Overcoming Worry and Anxiety
Dr Jerry Kennard

Physical Intelligence: How to take charge of your weight
Dr Tom Smith

The Self-Esteem Journal
Alison Waines

Ten Steps to Positive Living
Dr Windy Dryden

Transforming Eight Deadly Emotions into Healthy Ones
Dr Windy Dryden

Treating Arthritis: The drug-free way
Margaret Hills and Christine Horner

Treating Arthritis: The supplements guide
Julia Davies

Understanding Yourself and Others: Practical ideas from the world of coaching
Bob Thomson

When Someone You Love Has Depression: A handbook for family and friends
Barbara Baker

Overcoming Common Problems

Living with Hearing Loss

DR DON McFERRAN,
LUCY HANDSCOMB
and
DR CHERILEE RUTHERFORD

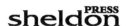
sheldon **PRESS**

First published in Great Britain in 2014

Sheldon Press
36 Causton Street
London SW1P 4ST
www.sheldonpress.co.uk

British Library Cataloguing-in-Publication Data
A catalogue record for this book is available from the British Library

ISBN 978-1-84709-272-4
eBook ISBN 978-1-84709-273-1

Typeset by Fakenham Prepress Solutions, Fakenham, Norfolk NR21 8NN
First printed in Great Britain by Ashford Colour Press
Subsequently digitally printed in Great Britain

eBook by Fakenham Prepress Solutions, Fakenham, Norfolk NR21 8NN

Produced on paper from sustainable forests

This book is dedicated to
Sam and Ben McFerran,
Zoe Handscomb-Williams,
and
Ben and Elle Van der Westhuizen

Contents

List of figures and tables

Note to the reader

This is not a medical book and is not intended to replace advice from your doctor. Consult your pharmacist or doctor if you believe you have any of the symptoms described, and if you think you might need medical help.

1

Introduction and definitions

Hearing is one of the five classical senses, the others being vision, smell, taste and touch. This is a simplistic view of the human body and there are actually many other senses, including balance, proprioception (awareness of the position of our joints), thermo-reception (awareness of temperature), pain and numerous more. Nevertheless, hearing is certainly one of our most important senses. Scientists will explain that the chief function of hearing is survival: hearing is there to pick up small danger signs in our environment – the sound of a predator creeping up on us or, in the twenty-first century, the sound of an approaching car as we cross the road. We still use the warning aspect of sound in our everyday lives: we have alarm clocks that use sound to wake us from sleep; we have smoke detectors in our buildings that use sound to warn us of fire; we fit our emergency vehicles with noisy sirens. But hearing offers us much more than that. Hearing has enabled us to develop speech as a form of communication. It has allowed us to develop sound as a form of enjoyment – music features in every human culture. Sound allows us to attend the pleasurable noises of nature: the babbling of a brook, birdsong, ocean waves.

Hearing range

Human hearing has an extraordinary range, from being able to hear the tiny sound of a whisper to being able to briefly tolerate a sound that is 100 trillion times louder than the threshold of hearing (that is, a range of 100,000,000,000,000). So the auditory system has to possess extraordinary sensitivity but also enormous resilience.

Sound definitions and measurements

There are various ways of measuring sound and describing it. One of the most important aspects of the sound is its level, and you will come across terms such as 'loudness', 'sound pressure' and 'intensity', all of which have specific meanings for an audiologist or scientist. These are words and phrases that are also used in everyday life and in this situation the definition is much less precise. Similarly you may see the unit of sound level, the decibel, written as dB, dB HL, dB A, dB SPL and in other ways. These distinctions are important from the scientific viewpoint but unimportant in the context of this book. We will use simple dB throughout the book to represent the level of a sound and use words like 'loudness' and 'intensity' in their everyday rather than scientific form. We apologize if this imprecision offends some readers. Approximate sound levels of various everyday sounds are shown in Table 1.1.

The tone or frequency of sounds is also important and this is measured in Hertz, which is the same as the more old-fashioned 'cycles per second'. Hertz is usually abbreviated to Hz. The frequency range of human hearing goes from a few Hz, which is very low pitched, to approximately 20,000 Hz, which is extremely high

Table 1.1   Some common sounds and their approximate decibel (dB) levels

Sound level (dB)	Example of sound
140	Close to a jet engine
130	
120	Thunder immediately overhead
110	Maximum output of some MP3 players
100	Circular saw
90	
80	Busy street
70	
60	Conversation
50	
40	Typical room
30	
20	Whisper or rustling leaves
10	Quiet breathing
0	Threshold of hearing

pitched. This range is seen in young people but high-frequency hearing does tend to reduce with age.

Hearing is commonly represented graphically on a chart called an audiogram (see Chapter 5 for details of hearing tests). This chart is somewhat confusing at first glance: the y axis of the chart depicts the hearing level and covers a range from –20 to +120 dB, but the biggest number is at the bottom of the chart. Furthermore, on an audiogram 0 dB does not mean absence of sound: by convention, 0 dB is the quietest sound that young people with normal hearing can hear 50 per cent of the time. Some people have better than average hearing, hence the negative numbers at the top of the chart: hearing at –20 dB is very good hearing, not bad hearing. The x axis of the chart shows the frequency of the sound that was used for the hearing test. Low-pitched sounds are at the left of the chart, with most standard hearing tests starting at 250 Hz and going up to 8,000 Hz, which is a high-pitched sound. A blank audiogram is shown in Figure 1.1.

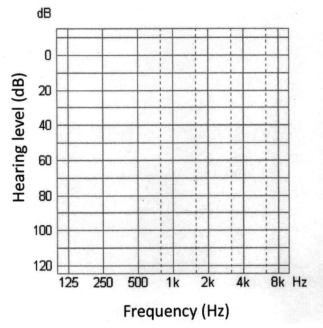

Figure 1.1 A blank audiogram

If people develop a hearing loss, the quietest sound that they can hear has a larger dB, but this is represented lower on the audiogram. So, good hearing is at the top of the audiogram and, broadly speaking, the lower the results on the audiogram, the worse the

Table 1.2 Various levels of hearing loss and their impact on speech perception

Hearing level (dB)	Hearing category	Impact
–20 to 25	Normal	Normal
26 to 40	Mild loss	Difficulty hearing speech in noisy environments
41 to 70	Moderate loss	Difficulty hearing normal speech even in quietness
71 to 90	Severe loss	Need hearing aids to hear speech
91 or greater	Profound loss	Great difficulty hearing speech, even with hearing aids

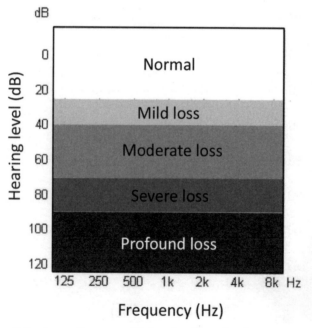

Figure 1.2 An audiogram with levels of hearing loss superimposed

hearing. Hearing losses are sometimes subdivided into normal, mild loss, moderate loss and profound loss. The exact levels of these definitions are not completely standardized but one commonly used system is shown in both tabular and graphical formats (Table 1.2 and Figure 1.2).

The sounds that are encountered during normal conversation can be superimposed on an audiogram, producing something that is called a speech banana (Figure 1.3). If your hearing test results are above the speech banana, you will probably be able to hear well. Conversely, if your hearing test results are below, you are likely to have a degree of hearing problem.

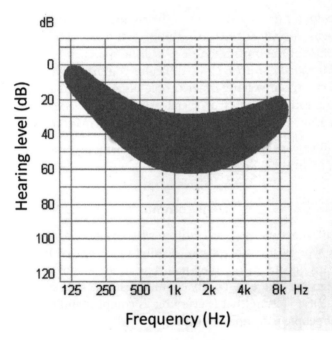

Figure 1.3 An audiogram with the range of common speech sounds superimposed, producing a 'speech banana'

Hearing loss terminology

We have chosen to entitle this book *Living with Hearing Loss* but other terms, such as 'hearing impairment', 'deafness' or 'being hard of hearing' are interchangeable with 'hearing loss'. There is no standardization in terminology and none of these terms is perfect. For example, if you were born without hearing you may understandably feel that you do not have hearing loss, because you never had any hearing and therefore there was nothing to lose. However, one area where there is standardization is the definitions of 'impairment', 'activity limitation' and 'participation restriction'. These have been formally defined by the World Health Organization with regard to hearing:

- *Impairment* is any reduction in the auditory function.
- *Activity limitation* refers to things you have difficulty doing because of the impairment, e.g. hearing speech.
- *Participation restriction* is the difficulty you may have taking part in activities involving other people because of the impairment, e.g. meetings, classes or social events. Not everyone with an impairment will necessarily experience participation restrictions.

We will discuss how hearing can affect many aspects of people's lives later in the book.

Deaf community

You will sometimes see Deaf written with a capital D. This refers to people who were born without hearing or developed hearing loss very early in life, before they had time to learn spoken language. People in the Deaf community communicate via sign language and have a Deaf Culture that is every bit as complex and rewarding as that of people with normal hearing.

Solutions to hearing loss

There is great variation in the management of hearing loss. This is largely a reflection of the fact that no one with hearing loss has exactly the same loss and personal circumstances as any other person. Two people with seemingly identical audiograms may have very different hearing abilities in real-life situations. Individual hearing requirements also vary: one person with a hearing loss may simply wish to hear the television better, whereas another with a similar loss may have more complex needs, wanting to hear in meetings, lectures, church services, concerts and plays as well as accessing an array of electronic devices such as mobile phones and MP3 players. There is therefore no 'one size fits all' solution to hearing loss.

2

The auditory system
and how it works

The ear (peripheral auditory system)

The fleshy outer part of the ear is known as the pinna (see Figure 2.1). This connects via the ear canal, or external auditory meatus, to the eardrum or tympanic membrane. The pinna, ear canal and eardrum together constitute the *external ear* and their function is to collect sound and funnel it to the eardrum. The eardrum is attached to a tiny bone, called the hammer or malleus. The malleus is attached to another bone, the anvil or incus, which in turn is attached to a third bone, the stirrup or stapes. These three bones are collectively known as the ossicles and conduct sound vibrations from the tympanic membrane.

The ossicles are sited in a small air-filled chamber that obtains its air via a tube called the Eustachian tube that opens at the back of the nose. Two of the ossicles, the malleus and the stapes, are attached to tiny muscles, the tensor tympani and stapedius respectively (not shown on Figure 2.1 for clarity). The air-filled space, the three ossicles and the two small muscles constitute the *middle ear*. The smallest of the ossicles, the stapes, sits in an opening in the bony framework of the ear called the oval window and conducts sound through this opening into the *inner ear*.

Another opening in the bone of the ear, the round window, is covered by a flexible membrane. As the stapes moves inward it causes microscopic movement of the fluid in the inner ear, which in turn causes the round window membrane to move outward. The inner ear is subdivided into the cochlea, which deals with hearing, and the vestibular apparatus, which deals with balance. The fluid movement within the cochlea generated by the vibration of the stapes causes a thin flexible sheet called the basilar membrane to vibrate, with different parts of this membrane vibrating according to the frequency of the incoming sound.

Rows of cells called hair cells sit on this membrane. These cells have small rods of muscle protein projecting from their surfaces which look like hairs under high-powered microscopes and give the cells their name. There are two groups of hair cells: they are called inner hair cells and outer hair cells. The vibration of the membrane moves the protein rods of the inner hair cells and this mechanical energy is changed to electrical impulses by the cells. Small nerve fibres underneath the hair cells collect these electrical impulses and convey them to the brain. The outer hair cells are

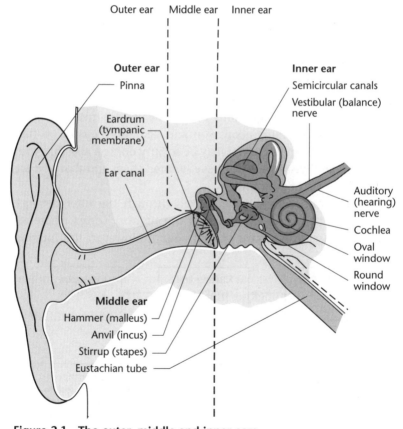

Figure 2.1 The outer, middle and inner ears

Source Adapted by kind permission of the Ear Institute, University College, London part of a complicated amplification system: small incoming sounds cause the outer hair cells to contract and expand, which makes the adjacent membrane vibrate more energetically. This causes a local feedback effect that enhances the activity of the inner hair cells and greatly improves the sensitivity of the cochlea.

Central auditory anatomy

The central auditory system is composed of several structures, some of which have imposing titles such as the inferior colliculus and the medial geniculate body. The names and anatomical descriptions of these structures are not very important in the context of this book. What is much more important are the functions that the central auditory system performs: these are depicted in Figure 2.2.

The first process is one of filtering and pattern recognition. This is something that we all recognize in our day-to-day life. It is the process by which the brain subconsciously decides what we are going to listen to and what can safely be ignored. For example, you can be standing in a busy party with lots of people talking around you, yet if one person mentions your name you are instantly aware that someone is talking about you and you will focus in on that conversation. Conversely you may be so busy doing a task that your friends or family say that you have ignored them and that you are in a little world of your own.

Sound information that is allowed through the filter network is passed to part of the brain called the auditory cortex where we become consciously aware of that sound. However, the filtering

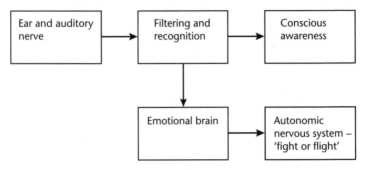

Figure 2.2   The various functional elements of the central auditory system

network can also pass this information to other parts of the brain, particularly something called the limbic system, which deals with our emotions. If you hear a sudden unexpected sound such as a creaking floorboard in the house at night, not only might you become aware of the sound but you may also become anxious about that sound. The emotional pathways in the brain can in turn activate other systems, particularly the sympathetic section of the autonomic nervous system. This is the body's fight-or-flight mechanism, the adrenaline centre. Thus, not only do you feel anxious but you also become more alert and your pulse goes up, your blood pressure goes up and you breathe slightly faster. If the creaking floorboard is caused by an intruder, these responses are very sensible and may even save your life. This example demonstrates the fact that the major function of your auditory system is to alert you and warn you about danger in your environment.

Of course, your auditory system is not just for protection: it also enables sophisticated communication via speech and produces many enjoyable sensations. Figure 2.3 shows the auditory system producing enjoyment by listening to a favourite piece of music.

The auditory system is also linked to other systems in the brain, particularly memory, and we are all familiar with the experience of hearing a particular sound, perhaps a piece of music from our past, which evokes a particular recollection. Furthermore, auditory events can trigger other responses in the body. For example, if we hear a sudden sound on one side we will automatically turn towards it in an effort to try and see the origin of the noise.

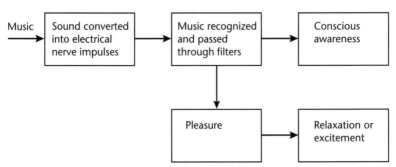

Figure 2.3   The central auditory system: processing and enjoying music

As we will see later in the book, hearing loss can occur owing to a problem in any part of this complex mechanism, ranging from blockage of the ear canal due to wax to perforations of the eardrum, conditions that stop the ossicles from moving properly, ageing of the cochlea and disorders of the auditory processing pathways of the brain. Problems within the cochlea are the commonest cause of adult hearing loss and it is widely assumed that this is due to damage to the hair cells. Hair cell loss is certainly a common cause of inner ear hearing loss but it is by no means the only cause: problems with the little nerve fibres can generate this type of hearing loss, as can stiffening of the cochlea's internal membranes or malfunction of the cells that deliver the cochlea's nutrition and maintain its electrical balance.

Ringing, buzzing, popping and cracking

Because the auditory system is so complicated and linked to so many other systems and processes within the body, it is probably inevitable that it periodically does things that we don't expect. Most people will have experienced brief periods when the hearing seems to go 'distant' for no particular reason. Similarly, most people will have had brief periods where their ears ring or buzz or whistle – sometimes at the same time as the hearing diminishes. These episodes are extremely common and are usually of no medical significance; doctors regard them as normal unless they are going on for more than five minutes at a time.

Likewise, when we yawn or swallow we open the pressure-balancing tube or Eustachian tube that runs from the back of the nose to the ear. We all do this many times each day and the opening of the tube generates a brief crack or pop in the ear. Generally we ignore this but some people focus on it and worry that it is something abnormal.

Feelings of blockage are common among people with inner ear hearing loss and/or tinnitus and such sensations may be misdiagnosed as wax, infections or malfunctioning Eustachian tubes. If these factors are not the reason for the symptom, what is the cause? We do not always find the cause but sometimes a blocked sensation is due to over-activity of the small muscles attached to the middle ear ossicles, the stapedius and tensor tympani. If these muscles contract continuously, the ear can feel blocked. This is sometimes known as tonic tensor tympani syndrome. In contrast, sometimes these muscles can contract rhythmically which can give rise to a fluttering sensation or buzzing noise in the ear. This is known as middle ear myoclonus. Such sensations can be very disturbing but are generally of no great clinical importance and do not signify that something is seriously awry. If you are worried about such symptoms, please mention them to your GP, audiologist or ear, nose and throat (ENT) doctor. Examination and a few simple tests such as audiometry and tympanometry (see Chapter 5) should exclude any significant underlying problem. An understanding of what is causing these symptoms is very helpful and frequently an explanation is the only treatment required.

3

Who has hearing loss and what other symptoms accompany hearing loss?

In this chapter we look at some of the facts and figures regarding hearing loss.

Overall prevalence of hearing loss

Determining the number of people with hearing loss is not an easy task but it is possible to reach some fairly broad conclusions. In the UK it is estimated that there are currently approximately 10 million people with at least mild hearing impairment – about 1 in 6 of the population. Scientists estimate that this figure will increase by about 14 per cent per decade as the UK population ages, reaching 14.5 million in 20 years' time. This represents a significant public health issue and the World Health Organization predicts that hearing loss will be one of the top ten health issues in the UK within 20 years.

Age and hearing loss

The majority of people with hearing loss are in the older age bracket, with 6.3 million out of the 10 million hearing-impaired people in the UK aged 65 or more. Just over 40 per cent of people aged over 50 years have some degree of hearing impairment. This figure rises to just over 70 per cent for those aged over 70 years and continues to rise with further age. The single biggest cause of hearing loss in the UK is age-related hearing loss, also known as presbyacusis.

Children

Congenital hearing loss is the most common birth defect in the Western world, with 1.6 of every 1,000 newborn babies having a moderate or greater hearing loss. Of these, in 0.6 per 1,000 the hearing loss affects one ear whereas in 1.0 per 1,000 the problem is bilateral. Among children born with hearing impairment, two-thirds have a genetic cause, and in 70 per cent of these children the hearing loss is the only birth anomaly. The single most commonly seen genetic hearing loss is caused by a defect in the gene that codes for a cellular protein called connexin 26. In the other 30 per cent of children born with genetic hearing impairment, the hearing loss is accompanied by abnormalities of other organs, including the heart, kidneys, eyes, skull or thyroid gland. A detailed discussion of the genetic syndromes that can be associated with congenital hearing loss is beyond the scope of this book but sources of further information that may be helpful are listed in the resources section at the end of the book.

Among the one-third of children born with hearing loss who do not have a genetic basis for that impairment, there are several common reasons: intrauterine infections such as cytomegalovirus, toxoplasma, herpes or rubella (German measles); premature birth and low oxygen during delivery; meningitis; some drugs given to treat serious infections in newborn babies, particularly a potent antibiotic called gentamicin. The last of these causes is particularly interesting as some people have an inherited sensitivity to gentamicin. A screening programme could potentially identify those babies that are at risk and ensure that they were given alternative antibiotics when necessary.

Some other cases of hearing loss develop after birth, and by the time children start school the number of children with permanent hearing impairment has risen from 1.6 per 1,000 to approximately 3.5 per 1,000. Overall, it is thought that there are around 45,000 children in the UK with a permanent hearing impairment. Although this is a small percentage of the total of 10 million people with hearing loss it is an extremely important subgroup. If children with hearing impairment are recognized early, steps can be taken to address the hearing loss using hearing aids, cochlear implants and educational support as appropriate and thereby improve their language acquisition, either orally or using sign language. Children with a permanent hearing loss are likely to do worse than their normal-hearing peers in the education system and are more likely to suffer from depression and other forms of mental illness. Early detection helps to address these issues.

Temporary hearing impairment is extremely common in childhood, particularly owing to a condition called otitis media with effusion (also known as OME, secretory otitis media or glue ear). Although this tends to cause a much less severe hearing loss it affects vastly more children than the congenital hearing losses discussed above: it is estimated that over three-quarters of children will have experienced one or more episode of otitis media with effusion by the age of 10 years. Most of these episodes are self-limiting and resolve spontaneously within a few days or weeks. A percentage of these episodes, however, do not resolve and result in persistent hearing impairment. Management of this condition is discussed in Chapter 6.

Gender and hearing loss

Although both men and women experience hearing loss, men are more likely to be affected, with approximately 1.5 times more men having a significant hearing impairment. This gender imbalance probably reflects more occupational exposure to noise among men, though men also tend to have more recreational noise exposure.

Noise exposure and hearing loss

Noise exposure does have a role to play in age-related hearing loss and the nature of that noise exposure is changing. People currently aged 70 or above may have experienced high levels of noise either in their workplace or during military service. Both of these forms of noise exposure are now recognized as being potentially harmful and, where possible, steps are taken to limit the exposure. Legislation regarding noise in the workplace now ensures that noisy machinery is acoustically treated or that operatives wear appropriate personal hearing protection (see Chapter 7). In military service, some noise exposure is probably unavoidable but the use of personal hearing protection has become widespread, at least during training, and the hearing of service personnel is now regularly monitored.

The area where noise exposure has increased recently is that of recreational noise exposure, particularly from music. The sound levels generated by personal music players such as MP3 devices can reach potentially injurious levels and there is fear that this will ultimately increase the prevalence of cochlear damage and hearing loss. There are relatively few scientific studies on this topic to date but those studies that are available suggest that we should indeed be more careful with these devices. Similarly, noise levels in night clubs and at concerts regularly exceed safe limits.

Seeking help for hearing loss

There is a huge delay between the onset of hearing loss and people obtaining help for that loss. Some studies have suggested that the gap between first noticing difficulty hearing and seeking help may be up to ten years. This is partly due to people not noticing or wanting to admit that they have a problem and partly due to the medical profession's habit of ignoring the symptom. One piece of research in the UK demonstrated that in over 40 per cent of cases GPs did not even arrange hearing tests when their patients complained of hearing difficulties.

Among the 10 million people in the UK with hearing impairments, it is estimated that approximately 6 million have hearing that could potentially benefit from the use of a hearing aid. The number of people who have been fitted with a hearing aid is 2 million. This is not an observation that is peculiar to the UK and many other countries have similar low take-up of hearing rehabilitation in general, and hearing aids in particular.

Conditions associated with hearing loss

There are some conditions that we would expect to be associated with hearing loss but there are some that are more surprising. The following is a discussion of some of the more common symptoms and conditions seen in conjunction with hearing impairment but is by no means an exhaustive list.

Tinnitus

Tinnitus is an awareness of a sound sensation that is not due to an external sound source. Tinnitus is extremely common, affecting 1 in 10 of the adult population, and although it is commonly assumed to be a ringing sensation, the sound perception can take almost any form, including buzzing, humming, whistling, white noise and occasionally even formed sounds such as music. It may be perceived in one or both ears or in the middle of the head or may even seem to be outside the body. Although tinnitus can occur in the presence of normal hearing, it is much more common in people who have hearing loss; when there is an associated hearing loss, correcting that loss is generally helpful in lessening the intrusiveness of the tinnitus.

Tinnitus is generated by a vicious circle in the central auditory pathways of the brain and is much more of a brain condition than an ear condition. Nevertheless, hearing loss is quite a potent trigger for generating tinnitus. Further details about the causes and management of tinnitus are discussed in another book in this series, *Living with Tinnitus and Hyperacusis* (see Further reading).

Disorders of loudness tolerance

Disorders of loudness tolerance are also very common among people with hearing loss. From first principles you might expect that as people's hearing deteriorates they would become more tolerant towards sound. This is not always the case, and one of the paradoxes of hearing impairment is that many people with a hearing loss are more, rather than less, sensitive to loud sounds.

The terminology for disorders of loudness tolerance is complex and still something of a work in progress. Hyperacusis is a condition characterized by dislike of all sounds above a certain level. Recruitment is a condition in which the dynamic range of people's hearing is compressed – in other words, they go from the impression that sounds are too quiet to the feeling that they are excessively loud with relatively little change in the intensity of the sound. This form of loudness intolerance is very common in people with cochlear hearing losses such as presbyacusis (see Chapter 6) and can result in difficulties fitting them with hearing aids. Misophonia is a dislike of certain particular sounds, also sometimes known as Selective Sound Sensitivity Syndrome or Soft Sound

Sensitivity Syndrome. Phonophobia is a particular form of misophonia in which the person is afraid or phobic of particular sounds.

Detailed discussion of the treatment of reduced loudness tolerance is beyond the scope of this book. However, one common feature seen in people with reduced loudness tolerance is that they often adopt what psychologists call fear-avoidance behaviour: they find sounds unpleasant and therefore they avoid them. At first glance this seems like a sensible strategy but it is often counter-productive. When people cut themselves off from sounds, the central auditory system in their brain notices that everything is quieter than previously and tries to rectify this by increasing central auditory gain. In effect this is 'turning up the volume knob'. This in turn makes the hearing more sensitive, which worsens the loudness intolerance. Although it initially sounds counter-intuitive, one of the most frequently used techniques for improving reduced loudness tolerance is to slowly reintroduce sound into the person's life. As with tinnitus, the management of hyperacusis is discussed in greater detail in the sister volume to this book, *Living with Tinnitus and Hyperacusis* (see Further reading).

Dizziness

Dizziness is another common symptom that may accompany hearing loss. Conditions affecting the inner ear can cause some specific types of dizziness, and this may happen in isolation or in association with hearing impairment. The dizziness that is due to inner ear problems is often characterized by vertigo. Vertigo is not, as is commonly assumed, a dislike of heights – the correct name for that is acrophobia. The medical definition of vertigo is that it is a hallucination of movement. People with vertigo feel that they or their environment is moving, often with a spinning sensation. Conditions such as Ménière's disease that feature both hearing loss and vertigo are discussed in Chapter 6.

Earache and discharge

Earache and discharge are sometimes seen in association with hearing loss, and if these symptoms are present infection is the likely cause. You may sometimes come across the medical names for these symptoms: 'otalgia' is medical-speak for earache, while 'otorrhoea' means discharge from the ears.

Dementia

It may surprise some readers to learn that dementia is more common in people with hearing loss. This association has only been recognized relatively recently and there are still a lot of unanswered questions about the link. It is not yet clear whether one condition triggers the other, whether they are caused by similar disease processes or whether the connection is purely coincidental. Research in this area is very much in its infancy and we still do not know if using hearing aids or other forms of hearing rehabilitation can help to prevent or delay dementia. Trying to correct an associated hearing loss, however, does seem a simple step to take to try and ameliorate this upsetting and difficult-to-treat condition.

4

Effects of hearing loss

Back in the eighteenth century, Dr Samuel Johnson (famous for his creation of the first English dictionary) described deafness as 'the most desperate of human calamities'. It might be argued that today, with hearing aids and cochlear implants available, the situation for hearing-impaired people is far less bleak. Nevertheless, there is much evidence to suggest that deafness can still have a distressing effect on people's lives.

Following the Second World War, a psychologist named Donald Ramsdell worked with soldiers who had lost their hearing in battle. Based on his interviews with them, he later described three levels of hearing which he called 'social', 'warning' and 'primitive'. He explained that we use our hearing at the social level to communicate with people around us and at the warning level to identify auditory signals that something is about to happen (like footsteps approaching or a door opening). Hearing at the primitive level is happening all the time; it is our sometimes barely conscious awareness of environmental sounds such as the hum of traffic or leaves rustling in the wind. Ramsdell made the point that all three levels contribute to our sense of self. Emphasis is often placed on communication, but he noted that people with hearing loss also describe feeling anxious about missing warning sounds ('Did I miss the doorbell?' 'Is it safe to cross the road?') and feeling cut off from the world because of not hearing music, birdsong or the general hubbub of daily life.

It is perhaps because hearing loss affects so many aspects of life that it can have such far-reaching consequences. Surveys carried out by the charity Hearing Link in 2005 found that rates of depression were almost five times higher among deafened people (those who have lost all hearing) than among the general population, and anxiety was two and a half times more prevalent. Other studies have also found evidence of psychological distress, loss of confidence and low self-esteem among people with hearing loss. Researchers

Patricia Kerr and Roddy Cowie conducted in-depth interviews with hearing-impaired people and found that, as well as communication problems, feelings of isolation and a deep sense of loss were also reported. For some people, losing hearing means losing your identity, because you are no longer able to contribute to conversation or take in information in the way you once did. Previously outgoing people can become withdrawn. Several deafened people have likened hearing loss to bereavement. Particularly if the loss is sudden or severe, it is not unusual to go through a grieving process which may include disbelief, sadness and anger.

Of course, deafness does not affect individuals in isolation. Relationships can come under severe strain when ease of communication is lost, and people with hearing loss can feel left out of family life. One complaint often made is that conversation becomes more functional; because communication is difficult, people restrict themselves to saying only what is necessary, and much of the 'banter' that goes on over the dinner table is lost. Friends may stop getting in touch when communication becomes so much more of an effort than it once was, and it may become more difficult to engage in social activities. All this can contribute to feelings of isolation and sadness.

Several studies have investigated the effects of deafness on relationships. British researchers Brooks, Hallam and Mellor interviewed people with hearing loss and their 'significant others' (most of whom were spouses) and found that both halves of the partnership reported similar levels of frustration, annoyance and embarrassment and both resented the reduction in social activity brought about by one partner's deafness. There was also frequent mention of annoyance over TV volume (too loud for one, too quiet for the other). Since most of the population in the Western world watches some TV every day, this has quite significant implications for the quality of daily life.

There may also be quite important changes in family dynamics when one person loses his or her hearing. People with hearing loss are three times more likely to be unemployed than people without a disability, so loss of income is a real difficulty for some families. It may be that roles are switched and the person with hearing loss can no longer be the main breadwinner. Roles can shift in more subtle ways, too; if the deafened person used to be the phone-call maker or the one who attended the school meetings, this may have to change, and such changes can unsettle the whole family.

The stigma that still seems to surround hearing loss does not help matters. Perhaps because it leads to misheard words and misunder-standings, deafness can be associated with stupidity in a way that other disabilities are not. Other people's intolerance of your dif-ficulty keeping up with conversation can further increase distress.

Nevertheless, the situation is not entirely bleak. People do adapt to hearing loss and many forms of rehabilitation are available, which will be discussed later in this book. It is not inevitable that the worse your hearing is, the worse your quality of life will be.

Some research has found that people with lower levels of hearing do not necessarily report a lower sense of well-being, but that there is a connection between well-being and the extent to which hearing loss is perceived to restrict life. Older age, having experience with hearing aids and having a good sense of humour are all factors that increase well-being for people with hearing loss. The good news is that, while the actual level of your hearing loss can probably not be changed, the extent to which it restricts your life can be.

Finally, there are some upsides to hearing loss. A Welsh professor of audiology, Dai Stephens, who had hearing loss himself, spent much time interviewing people about their experience of hearing loss and noted a number of positives, including less disturbance from neighbours' noise, being able to get out of disliked tasks such as making awkward phone calls, and also becoming more patient and more observant.

In short, losing hearing can be distressing, but it doesn't have to stay that way.

5

Diagnosis

Medical

In the UK, where vision is concerned there are formal NHS recommendations that everyone should have their eyesight tested at least once every two years. There is a programme for testing the hearing of children but there are no recommendations for checking hearing in adults. Seeking a hearing test is very much left to the individual. Some people with hearing loss recognize that they have a problem and actively seek help; many others feel that their hearing is satisfactory and it is their friends and family who have persuaded them that they should have their hearing checked.

Once you have decided that you should have a hearing test there are two main options: visit a private hearing aid dispenser or go through NHS channels. Most people in the UK obtain help for their hearing loss through the NHS. Private services are discussed later in the chapter.

People you may meet in the NHS

General practitioner

In the UK, the first step towards obtaining help via the NHS if you suspect you have a hearing loss is to discuss the matter with your general practitioner (GP) or family physician. Your GP will know the local arrangements for dealing with hearing loss and may refer you to an audiology or ear, nose and throat (ENT) department straight away. Alternatively he or she may be able to arrange for a hearing test to be done within the surgery, using either normal audiometric equipment or a small screening device. GPs can also treat those cases of hearing loss that are associated with infections or blockage of the ear by wax.

People in the UK cannot refer themselves directly to an NHS audiology or ENT department and require a letter of referral from their GP. This is in contrast to many other countries, where direct access is feasible. However, most UK audiology departments will take referrals directly from the GP for selected patients without having to go through the ENT department. This direct referral service is generally open to adults who have a stable, symmetrical hearing loss without other symptoms such as pain, ear discharge, troublesome tinnitus or dizziness. If you do not meet these criteria, your GP will refer you to the ENT department so you can have a full medical appraisal in addition to audiological assessment.

Audiologist

Audiology departments are staffed principally by audiologists, who are healthcare professionals trained to perform tests of hearing and balance. They also fit hearing aids and supply advice and counselling regarding hearing loss. There is some subspecialization in most audiology departments, with some audiologists focusing on children's hearing whereas others concentrate on balance issues or tinnitus.

ENT surgeon or audiovestibular physician

If your hearing problem does not meet the criteria for direct referral, your GP will refer you to a hospital-based doctor. In most areas this doctor will be an ENT surgeon: a doctor who has been trained in disorders of the head and neck and who carries out surgical operations. Most ENT surgeons have a subspecialism interest: some will be interested in conditions of the nose and sinuses; some will concentrate on ENT conditions in children; some will deal with tumours of the head and neck; some will specialize in conditions of the ears. The latter group are sometimes known as *otologists*.

If you have one of the specific medical conditions that are associated with hearing loss (Chapter 6), your ENT surgeon may suggest you undergo a surgical operation. This is relatively unusual for people with hearing loss and the vast majority do not need surgery. In a few areas your GP may refer you to a doctor called an audiovestibular physician (or audiological physician) rather than an ENT surgeon. These are doctors who have received subspecialism training in conditions of the auditory and balance system but unlike ENT surgeons they do not perform surgery.

The role for most doctors with regard to hearing loss is to take a medical history, examine the person and arrange further tests and investigations. Once the diagnosis is clear, most doctors then refer the person with hearing loss on to other members of the team for treatment.

Hearing therapist

Hearing therapists are healthcare professionals based in audiology departments who have trained to provide a rehabilitative service for people with all types of audiological problem. They can offer support to people who are distressed by hearing loss and undertake tasks such as helping people to overcome practical and emotional barriers to using hearing aids effectively and teaching communication skills. Hearing therapists demonstrate and offer advice about assistive listening devices (Chapter 10). They also help people who have other symptoms, such as tinnitus, in association with their hearing loss. Unlike audiologists they do not generally perform hearing tests or fit hearing aids. The career structure for staff in audiology departments in the UK is currently being restructured and the above job descriptions may alter over the forthcoming years.

Nurse specialist

In some audiology departments specially trained nurses offer an aural care service, delivering treatments such as wax removal, cleaning ears after mastoidectomy surgery (see Chapter 6) and treating ear infections.

Other healthcare professionals

Occasionally people with hearing loss need to see healthcare professionals, particularly if they have other symptoms in addition to the hearing problem. For example, people with significant tinnitus may be referred to a clinical psychologist, while those with dizziness and balance problems may be referred to a physiotherapist.

People you may meet outside the NHS

In the UK and most other countries, it is possible to visit to a private hearing aid shop. This may be a stand-alone business or it may be situated within a larger company such as an optician or pharmacy. No GP assessment or letter of referral is required: it is simply a question of contacting the shop and asking for an appointment.

A member of staff will then test your hearing and advise you as to whether or not you would benefit from a hearing aid. You will also be asked a detailed set of questions aimed at picking up serious ear disease, and if there is any suggestion that there is something more than wear and tear it will be suggested that you should contact your GP or ENT doctor. The member of staff who undertakes this may be an audiologist or may be a registered hearing aid dispenser. In the UK, hearing aid dispensers by law must be suitably qualified and registered with the Health and Care Professions Council (HCPC). In the interests of brevity, for the remainder of this book we are going to stick with the term 'audiologist' to denote any healthcare professional who performs hearing tests and fits hearing aids.

The ENT or audiovestibular physician appointment

The clinician in the outpatient clinic will ask not only about your tinnitus and hearing but also about your general health, current medication, allergies and employment history. If the doctor suspects that there is a genetic cause for your hearing problem, you may be asked whether any close relatives have or had hearing problems. The doctor will then perform a clinical examination. This will include examination of the outer ear, ear canal and eardrum using an otoscope (also known as an auroscope), which is a battery-operated light with a magnifying lens. If this reveals that your ears are infected or blocked with wax or debris from an infection, the doctor may want to examine your ears in more detail under a microscope and carefully remove the blockage.

The doctor may also examine other areas of the body, particularly the nose and back of the throat. This is because problems in this area can affect the Eustachian tube and cause conditions such as glue ear (see Chapter 6). This examination may just employ a light, a tongue depressor and a nasal speculum (a device looking a bit like sugar tongs that the doctor holds gently against the nostrils). If the doctor feels a better examination of the Eustachian tube openings is required, a flexible endoscope may be passed through the nose. This is a slightly uncomfortable but very quick examination, usually lasting about a minute. A local anaesthetic spray can be administered to the nose if necessary but in most cases this is not needed.

If your hearing problem is accompanied by other symptoms, such as dizziness, a much more in-depth clinical examination will be performed. Hearing tests will then be arranged, though in some units these are done before you see the doctor.

The audiology appointment

The audiologist will perform a series of tests to assess your hearing and auditory functioning. He or she will repeat the doctor's examination of ear and ear canal using an otoscope to ensure that the ears are clear and the test equipment will work effectively. This is usually followed by tympanometry, a procedure that involves holding a soft plastic probe against the ear or within the outer part of the ear canal. This apparatus gently puffs some air into the ear canal to check how effectively the eardrum is moving and detect whether the middle ear is functioning properly. Tympanometry can detect fluid under the middle ear and is particularly useful in the diagnosis of glue ear and some other forms of conductive hearing loss (see Chapter 6).

Next up is the hearing test, which in most cases is a test called a pure tone audiogram, often abbreviated to PTA. This is usually conducted in a soundproofed room or booth. Some people find the booths somewhat claustrophobic; if you are one of these people, please tell the audiologist – there will almost certainly be a less claustrophobic alternative.

The test involves the placement of headphones on the ears or sometimes earphones inserted into the ear canals. The headphones are connected to a machine called an audiometer, though nowadays this is often a computer with some boxes attached. This machine produces a range of tones, covering low to high-pitched sounds. The frequencies that are usually tested are 250 Hz, 500 Hz, 1,000 Hz, 2,000 Hz, 3,000 Hz, 4,000 Hz, 6,000 Hz and 8,000 Hz, which covers five octaves. Most audiometers can produce lower tones than this but these tones start to stimulate the body's vibration sensors as well as hearing, making the results difficult to interpret. Some audiometers can also produce higher-pitched tones which are used in some specialized hearing tests.

The audiologist will play the tones briefly and in a random fashion. You need to indicate when you can hear a sound by pressing a button. The purpose of the test is to establish a threshold of hearing or, in other words, the softest sound that you can possibly hear. People having a hearing test often comment that the sounds are very faint and they worry that they will have missed some. Please do not worry: because the test is determining the softest sound you can hear, the sounds are meant to be faint and the test procedure takes account of people missing some of the tones.

Sometimes the test also involves the presentation of a rushing noise to one ear, while still listening to the beeps. This is called masking and allows us to test each ear individually. This stage of the hearing test examines all parts of the hearing system and produces what are known as *air conduction thresholds*.

The audiologist may then place a little box against the bone behind the ear, held in place with a tight headband. This can be slightly uncomfortable but the box has to be in good contact with the bone. Sound energy is then played through the little box and into the bone. This sound goes directly through the bone to the cochlea and bypasses the ear canal, eardrum and ossicles. This produces information called the *bone conduction thresholds*, and comparing these to the air conduction thresholds enables us to work out whether a hearing loss is caused by the inner ear or the sound conduction structures in the outer and middle ear. While bone conduction is being tested, masking sound will usually be played into the opposite ear through a headphone. It is important that the hearing test is as accurate as possible, partly to enable an accurate diagnosis to be obtained and partly because the results are used for programming hearing aids if subsequently required. The results are plotted on a graph called an audiogram (see Chapter 1).

People sometimes comment that hearing beeps through a set of headphones in a soundproofed cubicle is not a very real representation of what their hearing has to do in the real world. We agree! However, it is fairly quick, simple, reproducible and standardized and, as we have already mentioned, it gives the necessary figures for programming the miniature computer in a digital hearing aid. There are some tests that try and give a more realistic view of how someone is hearing in everyday life, using methods called speech testing or speech-in-noise testing. These tests involve listening to words or sentences over headphones or via a speaker system and repeating what you have heard. For the speech-in-noise test there will be some form of background noise as well as the test words. This type of assessment can help the professional to prescribe different technologies, based on your individual results.

The clinician may also perform a test to check your uncomfortable loudness levels. This is a test where a series of tones are played and are gradually made louder and louder until you indicate that the next sound in the series is going to be uncomfortably loud. The test should never actually reach the painful stage and the output of the audiometer is limited so that it cannot cause permanent damage to the ears. This measurement is used to help to set hearing aids to ensure that the aids never amplify above your comfortable levels, ensuring your safety and comfort. If the thought of having this test worries you, please discuss it with your audiologist.

Your audiologist will next have a discussion with you and may use questionnaires to find out more about your life and how your hearing loss is impacting on it. This is a very important aspect of the appointment as hearing loss varies from person to person. Two people can have exactly the same documented hearing loss as indicated by their audiograms, but it can affect their lives in completely different ways. This is called a lifestyle assessment and will help the clinician to recommend the best course of action for you and your listening needs. Towards the end of the appointment your audiologist will summarize the results from all the assessments and make a few suggestions on how to best help you further. He or she may recommend hearing instruments or another treatment option, depending on your results. It is important that you participate in this discussion and feel free to discuss your preferences and any concerns that you may have at that point.

Further testing

A proportion of people with hearing loss will need further investigation, particularly if they have additional symptoms or if their audiogram shows a big difference between the two ears. The reason for performing further investigations is to make sure that there is no serious underlying cause for the hearing loss. The most common test that is required is a magnetic resonance scan (MRI). This produces detailed pictures of the auditory system, including the hearing nerves and adjacent brain. MRI scanners use strong magnetic fields and radio frequency energy to produce the pictures. To have an MRI scan of the auditory nerves takes approximately a quarter of an hour and involves lying on a machine. Initial MRI scanners had very confined interiors and many people worry that they are going to be put in a 'torpedo tube', but modern machines are much more open than previously and for an auditory nerve scan only the head goes into the scanner. The machine is still, however, slightly claustrophobic.

If you are worried about this, mention it to your doctor. It may be possible to administer a mild sedative for the time of the scan. The staff who operate the scanners are usually very good at dealing with people's fears and an intercom or panic button is available so you can contact them during the scan if necessary. MRI scanners are noisy, and it is usual to provide sound-attenuating ear defenders for the duration of the scan. Alternatively, sometimes it is possible to listen to music through headphones while the scan is being conducted (see Figure 5.1).

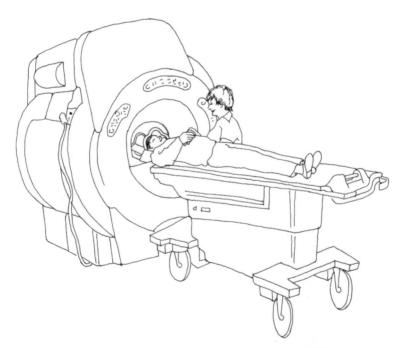

Figure 5.1 A patient undergoing a scan in a modern MRI scanner

Some hospital scanning departments administer an injection of a contrast medium which is a substance that highlights parts of the scan.

Not everyone can undergo MRI scanning: people with pacemakers or cochlear implants cannot go into the high magnetic field. People who have some types of metallic surgical implants are also excluded, though dental implants, dental fillings and orthopaedic implants such as artificial joints do not usually cause problems. It is usually safe to have an MRI scan if you have had cardiac stents inserted, but if you have any doubts at all please check with the scanning team before having your scan. There are some specialized scanners called open scanners or upright scanners that are much less claustrophobic than standard scanners, but you may need to travel a considerable distance to find one of these.

If you need a scan but cannot have an MRI or if you feel too claustrophobic even for the open scanner, there are alternatives. A computed tomography (CT) scan uses X-rays to produce similar pictures to MRI. CT scanning is much less claustrophobic, much quicker (usually only a matter of seconds), and much quieter than MRI. The trade-off is that the images produced by CT are slightly less detailed than MRI. CT does have one area where it is better than MRI: it is very good at showing the bone structure of the ear, and if the doctor suspects you may have a condition such as chronic otitis media (Chapter 6) he or she may choose to ask for a CT in preference to an MRI. For the few people who cannot be scanned by either MRI or CT, a specialized hearing test called brainstem evoked response audiometry (BSER or ABR) can be used to give more information about the auditory pathways.

Many people undergo these investigations, but the number who turn out to have significant pathology is very small: in our clinics, approximately 98 per cent of scans are normal. We tell our patients that we are not performing the scan because we think something is wrong: we are performing the scan to ensure everything is normal.

Occasionally doctors will arrange blood tests for people with hearing loss, particularly if the hearing deterioration has been rapid or if there are other associated symptoms. People who have dizziness as well as hearing impairment may require specialist tests called vestibular function tests. Once appropriate investigations have been completed, most people can be reassured that they do not have a specific underlying cause for their hearing problem. The small number who do turn out to have a specific medical condition are discussed in more detail in Chapter 6.

Investigating hearing loss in children

Testing the hearing of babies and children is challenging and developments in this area have been fascinating. Typically a variety of tests and methods are applied to obtain the best results and very often it may mean attending a series of appointments, particularly with babies and younger children. Because of differences in their development, different tests are selected based on the child's age and abilities. Clinicians will use a combination of case history information from parents, carers and educators, objective and subjective tests, and observations of the child to get to an accurate diagnosis. A cross-check principle is applied throughout the test battery as no single test will provide all the detail that is needed to document a child's hearing.

Neonatal screening

As we saw in Chapter 3, 1.6 in 1,000 newborn babies in the UK will be born with a hearing loss in one or both ears. Because of this, the parents of all newborn children in the UK are offered a hearing test for their child shortly after birth as part of an initiative called the Newborn Hearing Screening Programme. Similar schemes exist in many other countries. This test measures tiny sounds called *otoacoustic emissions* (OAE) that are produced by the ear in response to incoming sound, and is performed by putting a small probe in the baby's ear and connecting it to a laptop computer or dedicated otoacoustic emission test machine. The test is non-invasive and causes no discomfort.

Babies who do not pass the initial test are retested after an interval, and those who still do not pass are offered more detailed testing. The text test performed is usually one called *auditory brainstem response* testing (ABR). This test requires a baby to be in a settled, sleeping state. During this procedure the clinician places some small, self-adhesive sensors behind the baby's ears and also at the nape of the neck or high on the forehead. A series of sounds are then played into the baby's ears via tiny earphones that are specially designed for this type of testing. Although the presence of wires and sensor pads may look scary, the procedure is completely safe and pain-free and most babies remain sleeping while all of this takes place. If a baby wakes up during the process or becomes unsettled, the testing may have to be continued later. Sometimes it takes a few appointments to get all the results that are required, but it is important for subsequent management that accurate and reliable results are obtained.

If a baby is shown to have a significant hearing loss, he or she is referred to a multidisciplinary team (MDT) that includes ENT doctors, audiological physicians, audiologists, paediatricians, speech therapists, teachers of the deaf and representatives of the local sensory team. The MDT tries to ascertain the cause of the hearing loss, using a process called aetiological investigation. This process is extremely complex and involves tests that at first glance might appear to have nothing to do with the hearing: in addition to more detailed hearing tests, blood tests, scans and genetic testing, some unusual tests may be performed, such as an examination of the urine and an eye examination. Some children have additional tests such as an electrocardiogram (ECG or 'heart test') or an ultrasound scan of the kidneys. Urine is tested to check whether the baby has had an infection with a virus called cytomegalovirus (CMV). The other unusual tests may be performed if the medical team thinks that the hearing problem may be part of a wider genetic problem or syndrome that affects other organs in the body.

Depending on what the aetiological investigation shows, specific treatments may be given. The MDT then oversees the management of the hearing loss in all aspects, including education, speech therapy, provision of hearing aids and, where appropriate, cochlear implantation (see Chapter 9).

After the neonatal period, children in the UK have their hearing checked during a developmental check at two and a half years and then when they start school. If you think that your child has developed a hearing problem during this period, you should contact your GP. Parents are usually very astute at noticing changes in their child's hearing. Another factor that may point to a hearing loss is delay in speech and language development. There is considerable variation among children regarding their language skills but Table 5.1 lists what can be expected at various stages.

Table 5.1   Speech and language development at various ages

Age	Speech and language
12 months	Babbling and recognizing names of common objects
12 to 15 months	Speaking one or more words and able to follow a few simple, single-step instructions such as 'Please give me the ball'
18 months	20-word vocabulary
24 months	50-word vocabulary and putting two words together. Able to follow two-step instructions such as 'Please pick up the ball and give it to me'
2 to 3 years	Speaking in short sentences of three or more words

There is of course considerable variation among children, and divergence from this schedule of development does not necessarily imply that there is a problem.

Visual reinforcement audiometry

If a baby or toddler between the ages of 6 and 30 months requires a hearing assessment, this is typically performed using a procedure called visual reinforcement audiometry (VRA). The test is conducted in a specially designed soundproofed room equipped with toys and loudspeakers that are arranged in a particular way. The child will sit on a chair or on a parent or carer's lap, while one tester sits in front of the child, gently playing and showing her a toy. Another tester will operate equipment that produces a range of sounds from either the left- or right-side speaker in the test room. When the child hears the sound and turns her head in response to the sound, a light will come up above the speaker box and reveal an interesting toy such as a dancing toy animal. This is the child's reward for correctly turning her head when a sound was presented. This method of testing continues in the form of an auditory game, altering the pitch and loudness of the sounds until the clinician is satisfied that the results obtained are accurate and reliable. If the child becomes tired or loses concentration, affecting the accuracy of the results, a break will be offered or testing may continue at another time. With older children, the sounds can be delivered through insert earphones. Insert earphones are small foam tips that fit into the child's ear. This method allows each ear to be tested individually.

Play audiometry

Play audiometry is used for children from around the age of 3 years. The clinician trains the child to listen for a sound and, as soon it is heard, to perform an action like putting a wooden man in a boat or placing a ball on a stick. Once the clinician is satisfied that the child understands the game, he or she will continue to test each ear separately via headphones. The clinician may change the game or the toy to keep the child interested and motivated, but the principle stays the same – the child has to do something as soon as he hears a sound. The clinician will then plot the child's hearing levels on an audiogram and explain the results to the parents or carers.

Speech testing

Speech testing also forms an important part of the paediatric test battery and can give particular information about how a child hears different speech sounds. Different test methods are used at different developmental stages. One technique is to present the child with a range of items or pictures of items. The audiologist then asks the child to point to a particular item: for example, 'Show me the cup.' Sometimes these tests are run via automated, specially designed audio equipment, while at other times the audiologist uses his or her own voice to do the assessment. Increasingly, the test is carried out using a computer game.

6

Specific causes of hearing loss

In this chapter we will discuss the main causes of hearing loss. Where there is a specific treatment for a type of hearing loss we will describe it. We would, however, like to point out that it is easy to read the following descriptions of medical conditions and then imagine that you are going to have one of the more serious, such as Ménière's disease or an acoustic neuroma. Some of the conditions we are going to discuss, such as wax, glue ear and the hearing loss of ageing, are common. The majority of the other conditions are rare and will not apply to the majority of our readers.

Furthermore, there are a myriad of small-print causes of hearing loss, and to try and discuss them all is beyond the scope of this book. This chapter by necessity is an overview of some of the more common and some of the more clinically important causes of hearing loss. The only reliable way for you to obtain a diagnosis regarding your hearing loss is to have a proper medical consultation and appropriate testing. If you have a hearing loss and are in any doubt whatsoever about the cause of the loss, please discuss this matter further with your general practitioner or ENT doctor.

Types of hearing loss

Healthcare professionals divide hearing loss into three main categories – conductive, sensorineural and central. Conductive hearing losses are caused by problems in the outer or middle ear; in other words they are caused by a problem of the ear canal, eardrum or ossicles (see Chapter 2). Sensorineural hearing losses are those caused by problems in the cochlea or auditory nerve. Central hearing losses are hearing problems generated by the way that the brain processes the information that the ear has sent to it. None of these types of hearing loss are mutually exclusive: it is quite possible to have hearing loss that is due to two or even all three of these subtypes.

Another way of looking at hearing loss is to divide it into congenital and acquired: congenital hearing losses are those that are present at birth; acquired hearing losses develop after birth.

Conductive hearing losses

Congenital conductive hearing loss

A small number of people are born with abnormalities of their outer or middle ear. This may be the complete absence of a structure, or a particular part may be present but abnormal. For example, the ear canal may fail to develop or there may be a malformation of the ossicles. The treatment of this type of hearing loss depends entirely on the exact nature of the problem. It may involve reconstructive surgery, implant surgery, conventional hearing aids, bone-anchored hearing aids (Chapter 9) and general supportive measures.

Earwax

The skin of the ear canal produces wax – also known by its medical name, cerumen – as a protective measure. Many people worry that wax is somehow a harmful material, or they worry that their wax is different from other people's wax. There certainly are differences between different individuals' wax: some people produce dry flaky wax; some produce soft sticky wax; some produce hard wax; some wax is light in colour; some is dark. But these differences are largely genetically predetermined and just represent normal human variation such as the difference in hair or eye colour.

The ear has a way of cleaning itself that involves the skin of the eardrum constantly growing new skin cells which push the older cells to the edge of the eardrum and then down the wall of the ear canal. Doctors call this process skin migration and it brings wax, dirt and dead skin cells with it. Most ears left to their own devices get rid of their wax without needing syringing or the use of cotton buds.

Many ear symptoms, including inner ear hearing loss and tinnitus, can be accompanied by a feeling of ear blockage or fullness, and this leads many people to believe that wax is the cause of the problem. This blocked sensation is often something of a red herring and it is actually quite unusual for wax to be the sole cause of these symptoms. By all means get your ears checked, and if you are one of those people who regularly develops complete blockage of the ear due to wax then it is, of course, acceptable to get your general practitioner or ENT doctor to remove it. Most general practitioners offer ear syringing, though nowadays this uses an electrically powered pump rather than the traditional large metal syringe. Provided a few simple precautions are taken, ear syringing is a safe and effective procedure. Some people, however, find ear syringing unpleasant, while others have awkward-shaped ear canals that make it difficult to remove wax using this technique. ENT departments are equipped to remove wax by other methods, including the use of special microscopes, suction apparatus and delicate instruments. If you have a problem with regular wax build-up and dislike or are fearful of syringing, please ask to be referred to your nearest ENT department.

When wax does become important is when people with a hearing loss want to try hearing aids. If the audiologist fitting the aid needs to take an impression, the ear canal must be free of wax prior to the procedure. Once the hearing aid has been fitted, people who produce large amounts of wax may find that it tends to block the aid – they may therefore need to have it regularly removed.

Wax removal is not something that people can easily do by themselves and doctors see a regular stream of people who have damaged their ears by the use of cotton buds, matchsticks, ballpoint pens, knitting needles and hair grips! The old adage that the only thing to put into your ear is your own elbow is good advice. There are several proprietary gadgets available for sucking or washing wax out of the ear canal, but while some people may be able to use these effectively this is not a practice we encourage and we suggest it is much better to seek professional guidance.

Wax-softening eardrops are available from pharmacists, and some people find that using occasional drops can keep their wax under control. We recommend that if you want to try this you should discuss it with your general practitioner or ENT doctor before starting and should stick to the milder type of drops, such as olive oil or sodium bicarbonate drops. If you want to use olive oil, do buy medical drops from the pharmacy and not the culinary version, which may not be fully sterilized.

Recently there has been a growth of the use of ear candles to clear wax. Such candles have been implicated in several cases of significant damage to the ears and we strongly advise people to seek medical assistance rather than use these devices. In the USA the Food and Drink Administration (FDA) bans advertising that suggests ear candles have any medical use. Although this practice has been attributed to the Hopi tribe in the USA, representatives have gone on record stating that they are unaware of their tribe ever having practised ear candling.

Ear infections

Infections of the ear are divided into acute or chronic: acute infections have a sudden onset and are short-lived; chronic infections have gradual onset and a long or permanent duration. Examples of acute ear infections are acute otitis externa and acute otitis media.

Acute otitis externa is a common condition in all ages where the skin of the ear canal becomes inflamed and swollen. This results in itching, pain and discharge. If hearing loss is present, it is usually mild. It is more common in hot humid environments and can be triggered by scratching the ear canal with a fingernail or implement. Some people have a tendency to eczema of the ear canal which may predispose them to otitis externa. Treatment is usually with ear drops: these may be antibiotic ear drops, antiseptic drops, steroid drops or drops that combine antibiotics and steroids. Removing any debris in the ear canal is helpful as it allows the drops to penetrate: all ENT departments and some GP practices are able to do this. Strong painkillers may be required, and in severe cases tablet or injection antibiotics may also be needed. Although otitis externa is a one-off for most people, it can go on to become a chronic condition and in this situation it may be necessary to obtain an opinion from a dermatology doctor to check if there is an underlying skin sensitivity condition.

For many patients with chronic or recurrent otitis externa, one common risk factor is getting the ear wet. Therefore it is often helpful to try and keep the ear dry. This can be achieved by using cotton wool and coating the outside in Vaseline while bathing or showering. Alternatively, waterproofing earplugs or ear putty can be obtained from sports shops, pharmacies or via the internet. The ultimate form of waterproofing is to obtain moulded earplugs. These are sometimes called swim plugs and can be obtained from audiologists or hearing aid shops. The audiologist takes an impression from the ear canal in a similar way to making a mould for a hearing aid. The impression is then sent to a laboratory which manufactures the plug. Plugs can be supplied in a huge variety of colours and even with custom logos. Having brightly coloured moulds does make them harder to lose! Swim plugs, as their name suggests, can be used for swimming and they usually supply good waterproofing for surface swimming, though nothing will satisfactorily waterproof the ear for swimming underwater, snorkelling or diving. Swim plugs are also useful for chronic otitis media and people who have grommets in place (see p. 43).

Acute otitis media is another condition which is particularly common in childhood but can be seen at any age. Infection develops in the middle ear – the space underneath the eardrum. It often starts after a cold or flu and the infection usually reaches the middle ear via the Eustachian tube, which leads to the ear from the back of the nose. Pain rapidly increases, and if the infection is not quickly recognized and treated it can burst through the eardrum, causing a perforation. When this happens there is usually a blood-stained discharge. Hearing loss can be mild to moderate. Treatment is with antibiotics and painkillers. Nasal decongestants are also sometimes used, to encourage the Eustachian tube to work more effectively.

The classification of chronic otitis media is a fraught area where even the experts disagree. There are two main types: one is associated with holes in the eardrum or perforations; the second type is associated with the condition called cholesteatoma.

Perforations are most commonly caused by acute otitis media or trauma such as poking the ear with a pointed implement or being in the vicinity of an explosion. Most of the time acute perforations heal on their own, but occasionally this does not happen and the perforation persists. Sometimes these chronic perforations cause very little in the way of symptoms. On other occasions they can result in recurrent ear discharge and significant hearing loss.

If a perforation is not causing symptoms, it may not need any treatment at all, but if treatment is needed this is usually a surgical operation to repair the eardrum. This is called myringoplasty or tympanoplasty and uses the patient's own tissue to put a patch on or under the hole. The aim is to give an intact eardrum, which lessens the risk of further infections. It is a graft operation, and like all graft operations it does not always work. Hearing may or may not be improved and there is a very small risk that hearing could be worsened. If the surgeon finds that the ossicles have been damaged, he or she may try and repair them or replace them with synthetic bones: this is called ossiculoplasty.

Cholesteatoma is a condition in which the pressure-balancing mechanism of the ear malfunctions and part of the eardrum becomes sucked inwards, or in medical parlance becomes retracted. The retracted segment then traps dead skin cells which can develop a persistent low-grade infection. This in turn slowly erodes normal structures such as the ossicles and can even eat through the bone of the skull to carry infection towards the brain. Symptoms are often minimal until the condition is well advanced: a slowly progressive hearing loss and a scanty but smelly discharge may be the only symptoms. The potential seriousness of this condition, allied to the paucity of symptoms, is a further reason why people with hearing loss should seek medical advice. It is sometimes possible to keep this condition under control by regular inspection and cleaning of the ear in the ENT outpatient department. If this does not work, then surgery is required.

This is a very complex topic which could easily fill a book all on its own. The operation is usually some form of mastoidectomy but multiple other names are used, depending on exactly what is involved: radical mastoidectomy, modified radical mastoidectomy, atticotomy, atticoantrostomy, intact canal wall mastoidectomy and combined-approach tympanoplasty are all different types of mastoidectomy. The basic principle is to remove the retracted eardrum with any associated chronic infection, drilling away part of the bone of the skull for access. Once the disease process has been removed, the ear is reconstructed, using grafts as necessary. The aim of surgery is to make the ear safe and prevent infection reaching structures such as the brain; it is major ear surgery with significant potential risks. It is impossible to generalize with this type of surgery, and if you are going to have such an operation it is imperative that you have a full discussion with your surgeon of what is involved in your particular case.

With both types of chronic otitis media it is sensible to keep the ears dry, using one of the techniques described above, if surgery has not been undertaken. After surgery it may be possible to get water into the ears again. This is something else that you should discuss with your surgeon.

Glue ear

Glue ear is a very common condition which occurs predominantly in childhood but can affect people of any age. It is due to a build-up of fluid in the middle ear which prevents the eardrum and ossicles from moving properly. The fluid is sometimes thin and watery but on other occasions it is thick and stringy, hence the title of glue ear. There are several other medical names for this condition, including otitis media with effusion and secretory otitis media.

The main cause of glue ear is thought to be immaturity or malfunction of the Eustachian tube. If this tube does not function properly, air does not reach the middle ear to balance the pressure therein. The inside of the middle ear then reacts to this pressure imbalance by producing fluid. Other hypotheses have been suggested: one modern theory that is currently being researched is that glue ear is due to persistent low-grade infection caused by thin layers of bacteria called biofilms. Risk factors for glue ear include having enlarged adenoids or allergies. Parental smoking also increases the risk, even if the parents smoke outside the house. Having been breastfed appears to confer some protection.

Glue ear generally only produces a mild hearing loss, but as the condition tends to occur at an age that is in a critical period for language acquisition this mild loss can have a disproportionate effect on learning to speak, read and write. Diagnosis is by examining the ears, performing an age-appropriate hearing test and performing tympanometry (Chapter 5).

Brief periods of glue ear are very common and many cases resolve spontaneously. The first treatment is therefore usually to do nothing – just wait and retest, usually after about three months. If the problem persists after three months, active treatment may be needed, but only if the glue ear is causing significant problems with speech development or education. In some cases of glue ear, the hearing loss is so mild that treatment is unnecessary.

When treatment is necessary, the most common approach is to insert grommets. A grommet, also known as a ventilation tube, is a small flanged plastic or metal tube that is inserted under local or general anaesthetic into the eardrum. There is a hole through the middle of the grommet, thereby providing a connection between the ear canal and the middle ear. This allows air into the middle ear, bypassing the non-functioning Eustachian tube. Once the pressure has been equalized, the glue ear resolves.

The medical community is divided about how to look after grommets while they are in situ. Some doctors recommend keeping the ear dry whereas others feel this is unnecessary. The advice here is to check with your own ENT doctor.

Grommets are very safe but complications do sometimes happen. By far the commonest is developing an infection in the grommet. This usually responds well to treatment with antibiotic drops: oral antibiotics are usually less effective.

Eardrums are constantly growing and this growth slowly pushes the grommet back out again in a process that doctors call extrusion. When the grommets come out, in many cases the eardrums heal, the ear then works normally and no further treatment is needed. In a proportion of cases, the eardrums heal but the glue ear returns. In this case grommets can be reinserted. Occasionally the eardrum does not heal and a small hole or perforation remains. This can be treated just like any other perforation (see 'Ear infections', p. 41). People with grommets often ask if they can fly with grommets in situ: the answer is yes. In fact, the grommets automatically balance the pressure and make flight more comfortable than normal.

There are other possible ways of treating glue ear: temporary hearing aids can be fitted in the hope that the Eustachian tube will eventually sort itself out and start working normally. Decongestants or steroid sprays can be used in the nose to try and improve Eustachian tube function. Devices have been developed whereby the person with glue ear raises the air pressure in the nose using an electrically driven pump or special balloon. This increased pressure forces the Eustachian tube open and equalizes the pressure inside the ear. Such devices can be obtained at good pharmacies: ask your doctor or pharmacist for advice if you wish to try this option.

A new way of treating glue ear is currently being studied. This is at a very experimental stage and is not yet widely available. It involves a minor operation during which the surgeon looks at the opening of the Eustachian tube using a small endoscope passed through the nose. A very fine balloon is inserted into the Eustachian tube and inflated to stretch the tube and let it work more effectively. This technique is called balloon dilatation of the Eustachian tube.

Otosclerosis

Otosclerosis is an interesting condition in which some of the bone within the ear becomes thicker and develops a sponge-like texture. This process prevents the stapes or stirrup bone from moving properly and hence reduces the amount of sound energy passing from the eardrum to the inner ear or cochlea. Otosclerosis is partly due to genetic factors, so if you have a relative with this condition your own risk may be increased. However, there are also other factors at play: previous infection with measles virus seems to be one factor that increases the risk. In some cases the condition appears to be linked to hormonal changes, so women with otosclerosis may observe that their hearing worsens around the time of pregnancy. Whatever the exact cause of otosclerosis, the incidence seems to be decreasing and what used to be one of the common causes of hearing loss in young to middle-aged adults is now quite a rarity.

Simple examination of the ear and use of routine hearing tests usually gives the diagnosis. Treatment may be simply a question of waiting and retesting if the symptoms are mild. Hearing aids are often very helpful, not only with regard to the hearing itself but also with regard to any accompanying tinnitus. The use of fluoride tablets can help, though in the United Kingdom and many other countries this treatment is rarely utilized.

If these simple measures have not helped, an operation called stapedectomy or stapedotomy offers the chance of a cure. In this procedure the surgeon operates down the ear canal, makes a small incision and turns the eardrum forwards to reveal the ossicles or bones of hearing. If the diagnosis of otosclerosis is correct, the stapes will be immobile. The top portion of the bone is then removed and a small hole is created with a micro-drill or laser into the inner ear. A prosthetic bone (usually plastic or a mixture of plastic and metal) is inserted and the eardrum is returned to its normal position. Most surgeons insert a dressing in the ear canal for a period of several days following the surgery. Somewhere between 80 and 90 per cent of people experience dramatic improvement in their hearing following surgery, and if they also had tinnitus this is generally reduced or even abolished. There is, however, a caveat. As with any surgery there are risks attached to this procedure and the main risk is damage to the inner ear. Between 1 and 5 per cent of people have worse hearing after the surgery, and that may mean complete hearing loss. If you have otosclerosis and are contemplating surgery, you need to have a long talk with your surgeon and discuss outcome figures. Any surgeon who is regularly performing stapedectomy surgery should be able to tell you what his or her results are as opposed to quoting general figures for all ENT surgeons.

Sensorineural hearing losses

Congenital sensorineural hearing loss

Significant congenital sensorineural hearing loss affects about 1.6 in 1,000 newborn babies in the United Kingdom and there are a vast number of potential causes, including intrauterine infections, genetic factors, premature birth and birth problems such as starvation of oxygen during delivery. Of the genetic causes, some are associated with other medical problems and the child may have a medically recognized syndrome. The majority of genetic causes, however, are not associated with any other health problem. The most commonly discovered example of this type of sensorineural loss is an abnormality in an ear protein called connexin 26. A national programme was set up in 2001 in the United Kingdom with the aim of testing the hearing of every newborn baby shortly after birth; this has greatly improved the rate at which this type of hearing loss is detected. Similar schemes exist in many other countries. Congenital hearing loss is discussed in more detail in Chapter 3.

Presbyacusis

Presbyacusis (sometimes written as presbycusis) is the medical name for the hearing loss that is associated with ageing. It is extremely common in industrialized countries, affecting about 70 per cent of those aged over 70 in the UK (the prevalence of this type of hearing loss is discussed in more detail in Chapter 4). It is due to a mixture of genetic and environmental factors. A certain amount of wear and tear occurs due to exposure to noise and other agents such as industrial solvents and cigarette smoke. The rate at which this wear and tear happens is partly determined by one's genetic makeup. The human inner ear, in common with the ears of other mammals, has very limited powers of regeneration: once cells within the cochlea have died, the body cannot replace them. Thus the wear and tear gradually builds up during the lifetime of the individual. Many parts of the inner ear can be affected in this process, including the hair cells, nerve cells, internal membranes and the mechanism that delivers oxygen and nutrients.

Noise-induced hearing loss

People who are exposed to a lot of occupational or recreational noise tend to develop a predominantly high-frequency sensori-neural hearing loss that in many ways mimics an accelerated form of presbyacusis. This type of hearing loss is mainly due to damage to the outer hair cells in the cochlea.

Ménière's disease

Ménière's disease is a rare condition that is hugely overdiagnosed. There are many unanswered questions about Ménière's disease and the symptoms vary greatly from person to person. So far as it is possible to generalize, a typical Ménière's disease person first develops symptoms between the ages of 20 and 40 years. The symptoms come as attacks, and between attacks the person initially returns to normal. In a typical attack the person develops a sensation of blockage and tinnitus in one ear. Then after a variable length of time, the hearing goes down and the person becomes very dizzy, often feeling that everything is spinning around. After a period varying from half an hour to several hours the dizziness wears off and the other symptoms abate. The attacks may happen very infrequently or may be common occurrences. As the condition progresses over the years it is common for the person to develop a degree of permanent hearing loss in the affected ear in addition to the episodic fluctuations.

At the onset of Ménière's disease the most distressing symptom is the dizziness. With time, however, the dizziness frequently becomes less of a problem and this aspect of the Ménière's disease often seems to burn itself out. The hearing loss and tinnitus, by contrast, often become more evident later in the course of the condition. Ménière's disease usually only affects one ear, though there is a small risk of it going on to affect the opposite ear.

The cause of Ménière's disease remains an enigma. We think it is due to a periodic build-up of fluid in the inner ear that temporarily disrupts the hearing and balance organs. The reason for this fluid build-up is not known. In a few cases genetic factors seem to be involved, though this is rare.

Treatment usually starts with medication to suppress the dizzy attacks and people are often advised to adopt a low-salt diet. Such measures control the symptoms in the majority of cases. If control is not achieved, surgery may be required. Although a large number of surgical interventions have been tried in the past there are currently four techniques in widespread usage.

Grommet and pressure device

A grommet is inserted into the eardrum using the techniques described for glue ear (see p. 43). When a person feels that a Ménière's attack is coming on he or she holds a pressure device against the ear. This gently puffs air through the grommet into the middle ear, and this is thought to affect the inner ear pressure, thereby preventing the Ménière's attack from happening.

Endolymphatic sac decompression

This is an operation usually performed under general anaesthetic in which the bone behind the ear is drilled away until a portion of the inner ear called the endolymphatic sac is exposed. The thinking behind this operation is that if the bone covering the endolymphatic sac is removed, the sac can swell more easily and thereby take the pressure off the rest of the inner ear. Some surgeons insert a small 'shunt' tube into the sac as a further measure in controlling the pressure.

Vestibular nerve section

This is an operation usually performed under general anaesthetic. A small hole is created in the bone of the skull and then part of the brain is gently lifted out of the way to expose the hearing and balance nerves. The balance nerves are cut, leaving the hearing nerve intact. This is very effective in controlling the episodic dizziness but does not prevent the hearing from fluctuating.

Gentamicin injection

Gentamicin is an antibiotic that is given by injection for serious, potentially life-threatening infections. One of its side effects is that in high doses it damages the inner ear, particularly the balance part. This side effect of the drug can be used to control Ménière's disease by selectively destroying the balance function of the inner ear while retaining the hearing function. A small quantity of gentamicin is injected, either directly through the eardrum or through a previously implanted grommet, and diffuses into the inner ear.

All the treatments used in Ménière's disease are designed principally to help the dizziness. We have a reasonable idea of how they work in this respect. We have less evidence, however, in how they help hearing. Standard forms of hearing rehabilitation such as hearing aids can of course be used.

Acoustic neuromas

An acoustic neuroma is the commonly used name for a small benign tumour which grows on the nerve of hearing and balance. The correct medical name is vestibular schwannoma. The nerve of hearing and balance, which is also known as the vestibulocochlear nerve or the eighth cranial nerve, is formed of several different components, some carrying auditory information and some carrying balance information. Acoustic neuromas generally grow on one of the balance nerves, either the superior vestibular nerve or the inferior vestibular nerve. Apart from a few very rare cases which are associated with an inherited condition called neurofibromatosis II, the cause of acoustic neuroma remains unknown.

The vast majority of these tumours grow very slowly, enlarging by less than 1 mm per year; however, as they slowly enlarge, they press against the hearing part of the vestibulocochlear nerve. This eventually results in hearing loss. Tinnitus is a common accompanying symptom and occasionally can be the only symptom of an acoustic neuroma. Imbalance or dizziness can also occur. The best way of diagnosing an acoustic neuroma is by performing an MRI scan (this and other diagnostic techniques are discussed in Chapter 5).

Because many acoustic neuromas grow extremely slowly, if at all, many do not need active treatment. Many people with acoustic neuroma simply undergo regular (often annual) MRI scans to ensure that the tumour remains small. This option is sometimes called 'watch and wait'. If the tumour is larger when first detected, or seems to be a more rapidly growing type, active treatment may be needed. This may be some form of radiotherapy treatment or surgery. Surgical procedures for acoustic neuromas are much safer than they were 50 years ago but nevertheless this is still a major undertaking. Surgery is very effective at removing the tumour but some forms of surgery destroy any residual hearing in the operated ear. Some other types of surgery try and preserve whatever hearing is left, but this is just preservation and does not improve the hearing; hearing preservation surgery is not possible in every case. Similarly, with radiotherapy the best treatment outcome that can be expected is preservation of remaining hearing rather than an improvement. If a hearing preservation technique has been employed, a hearing aid can be tried if necessary.

Sudden sensorineural hearing loss

This is a form of hearing loss that comes on very rapidly, over a matter of hours or a day in comparison to the more usual forms of inner ear hearing loss which develop over months or years. Sudden sensorineural hearing loss can be caused by a large number of disparate conditions including viral infections of the inner ear, problems with the microcirculation of the inner ear and auto-immune diseases in which the body's own defences attack its own tissues. Frequently, however, the true cause remains a mystery.

Because it can have so many different causes the clinical course and outcome are difficult or even impossible to predict. Fortunately many cases of sudden sensorineural hearing loss recover spontaneously. Sudden sensorineural hearing loss is a medical emergency, and if your hearing does deteriorate very rapidly you should seek immediate medical advice.

Multiple treatments have been tried and many ENT departments have protocols for dealing with this condition. Steroid tablets are usually the mainstay of treatment. If the hearing loss does not respond to this treatment, some doctors recommend injections of steroids directly through the eardrum. Other drugs have sometimes been advocated to try and improve the blood circulation of the inner ear but there is little evidence to support their usage and some of them carry significant potential risks.

Central auditory conditions

There is a group of people who demonstrate hearing problems in real-life situations but for whom standard hearing tests show that their ears are working normally. In these people it is the auditory pathways of the brain that are the cause of the problem. This phenomenon was only recognized relatively recently and the terminology is still very confusing, with multiple names applied to conditions that at first glance seem very similar. Terms such as auditory processing disorder, central auditory processing disorder, obscure auditory dysfunction, King Kopetsky syndrome, auditory dyssynchrony, auditory neuropathy and auditory neuropathy spectrum disorder are all used.

Much remains to be learnt about such conditions, but one thing is clear – understanding hearing means that we have to consider neural pathways in the brain as well as the function of the ears. Some people prefer not to regard these conditions as being examples of hearing loss as the ears may be functioning completely normally. However, patients with such conditions present to medical practitioners and audiologists as if they have a hearing loss and we feel it is completely appropriate to discuss these problems in a book on hearing loss.

The best way to manage such conditions is still unclear. Speech therapy, occupational therapy, hearing therapy, educational interventions, computer-based auditory training programmes and the use of FM communication systems are all potential options. To further muddy the water in this already complicated area, it is quite possible for someone with a conductive or sensorineural hearing loss to also have a central auditory problem.

General health and hearing

Some forms of hearing loss, particularly sensorineural hearing losses, are influenced by other health issues. Some of these are things that we can do nothing about, such as ageing and our genetic makeup, but there are some other conditions and behaviours where we possibly can influence hearing loss. We have already seen that glue ear in children is more likely if their parents smoke. Unsurprisingly, glue ear is also more likely among adults who are smokers. Perhaps more surprisingly, smoking also increases the risk of developing sensorineural hearing loss. Some medical conditions such as diabetes and cardiovascular disease also increase the risk of developing sensorineural hearing loss. If you have one of these conditions, keeping it well under control may help to lessen the risk of developing hearing loss.

Caveat

At the end of this chapter we are just going to reiterate what we said at the start: please do not try and self-diagnose. We firmly believe that everyone who thinks they have a problem with their hearing should obtain an appropriate medical opinion and a hearing test from an appropriate professional.

7

Prevention

One obvious approach to dealing with hearing loss is to try and prevent it before it happens. Noise exposure is a major factor in causing hearing loss and limiting that noise exposure is an effective preventative measure. If you are reading this book because you already have a hearing loss, you might be tempted to ask whether it is too late to worry about hearing protection: are we asking you to close the stable door after the horse has bolted? We would argue that it is even more important to look after your hearing if you already have a loss. If your hearing is impaired, it is vital that you try to conserve whatever hearing you still have.

The most obvious way to reduce your noise exposure is simply to stay away from the noise. This may not be possible if the source of noise is your workplace. Alternatively, the noise may be associated with something you enjoy, such as music, riding motorbikes or recreational shooting. Fortunately there are ways to protect yourself in almost all situations such that you can continue being in the noisy environment.

Noise at work

Legislation

Most countries have laws governing noise exposure in the workplace. In the UK the current rules are contained in a document called the Control of Noise at Work Regulations 2005 which is based on a European Union directive. This document is freely accessible on the internet from the Health and Safety Executive; contact details are given in the resources section at the end of this book. As with most government documents, it is quite complicated. The basic principles, however, are fairly simple: three exposure levels are set, defining an average daily or weekly level of noise exposure and a peak exposure. These levels are defined in Table 7.1.

Table 7.1 Occupational noise exposure levels set by the Health and Safety Executive in the UK

	Average level of exposure (dB)	Peak sound pressure (dB)
Lower exposure level	80	135
Upper exposure level	85	137
Exposure limit	87	140

The methods of assessing the average and peak levels are complex but the regulations based upon these levels are reasonably straightforward. At the Lower Exposure Level employers have to assess the risk to employees' health and provide information and training. At the Upper Exposure Level employers have to provide a programme of noise control using methods such as the provision of hearing protection and defining hearing-protection zones. The third limit, the Exposure Limit, is the legal limit of noise beyond which workers should not be exposed. Another principle enshrined in the regulations is that employers have a duty to provide health surveillance of those employees exposed to sound at or above the Upper Exposure Level. The regulations also give simple guidelines to employers and employees to estimate when noise is likely to be a problem in the workplace: if you work in an area where you think noise levels exceed the levels described above, the first step is to discuss your concerns with your employer. The Control of Noise at Work Regulations only cover sound levels in the workplace and do not apply to recreational noise.

Identifying if your workplace is noisy

The following simple guidelines are reproduced from a Health and Safety Executive leaflet called 'Is your workplace noisy?' You will probably need to take some action if any of the following apply to you or your workers:

- You're surrounded by intrusive noise for most of the working day. Examples of intrusive noise from everyday life are a busy street and a vacuum cleaner.
- You have to raise your voice to be heard by someone just two metres away for at least part of the day.

- You use noisy powered tools or machinery for more than half an hour a day.
- You work in a noisy industry such as construction, road repair, engineering or manufacturing.
- Your work causes impacts such as hammering, drop forging, pneumatic impact tools, etc.
- You work with explosive sources such as cartridge-operated tools or detonators, or guns.

The leaflet also points out some noise exposure that is unlikely to be hazardous:

- Busy offices
- Shops
- Travelling in cars on motorways.

What to do if you think your workplace is too noisy

If you have used the above rules of thumb and think that your workplace is too noisy, the first step is to notify your employer of your concerns. In some companies there may be a trade union-appointed safety representative or other employee representative who may be able to help in this process. Depending on the size of your company there may be a company doctor or other occupational health professional who can assess your hearing level. Failing this, you should contact your GP who may be able to check your hearing or will be able to refer you to an audiology or ENT service. If you think your hearing may already have been damaged and you are thinking of taking legal action, this is discussed in Chapter 11.

Reducing noise at source

Many manufacturing processes use machinery that generates significant noise. It is often possible to engineer machinery in such a way that noise levels are minimized. All too often, however, noise levels from machinery are either ignored or treated as a minor factor in the choice of equipment: equipment costs and production rates are usually bigger drivers of choice. Machinery also tends to be noisier if it is not properly maintained, so a regular service schedule should be implemented.

Enclosing noisy equipment

If the use of noisy machinery is inevitable, the machine should be sited in such a way as to minimize its impact on employees. Acoustically absorbent screens and barriers should be installed to reduce the amount of noise reaching the people in the workplace.

Time limiting

Damage caused to the ears is not just a reflection of the noise levels that people are exposed to but also depends on the duration of exposure. If employees have to work in a noisy area, reducing the amount of time spent in the noisy environment is helpful. The same principles can be applied to recreational noise: breaking up noise exposure is just as helpful when that noise is generated by musical instruments.

Personal protection

Sometimes it is not possible or practical to use quiet machinery or to acoustically isolate it. In this case, providing people with ear protection is the next best option. Earplugs and earmuffs are the most commonly used devices and these are cheap and widely available. Earplugs may be compressible foam plugs which expand to fill the ear canal or pre-moulded plastic plugs. Some plugs are linked by a thin cord or plastic band. This makes the plugs harder to lose but makes little difference to the acoustic properties.

Manufacturers of hearing-protection devices quote figures for the amount of sound attenuation that the devices provide. These figures are obtained in laboratory conditions by people who are trained in the usage of the devices. Real-life figures suggest that these manufacturers' figures are often wildly optimistic. Broadly speaking, the earmuff protectors provide the best protection, with foam earplugs coming second and finally pre-moulded plugs. Personal ear protection equipment does have disadvantages: the devices are sometimes awkward or uncomfortable to wear, especially in conjunction with other safety equipment; they make the ear hot and sweaty; they increase the risk of infection of the ear canal. One issue seen with the earmuff pattern of protectors is that they may not fit properly if the person is wearing spectacles or safety glasses: the arm of the spectacles breaks the acoustic seal around the ear, allowing more sounds to enter the ear.

Ear protection devices also need to be looked after. Foam plugs should ideally be treated as single-use items. If you do reuse them, they should certainly be replaced if they become dirty or lose their elasticity. Moulded plastic plugs can be washed in soap and water and reused for up to a few weeks. The cushions of earmuffs can also be cleaned with soap and water. The cushions and foam inserts in earmuffs gradually deteriorate and this pattern of protective device should be replaced approximately every six months. If there is any obvious damage to any form of hearing-protection device, replacement should be immediate.

It is also possible to use active hearing protection or sound cancellation. This is a technique by which electronic circuitry is built into a set of headphones. The circuitry analyses the sound around the wearer and produces sound waves with the opposite phase to the ambient noise, cancelling out that noise. This is a useful technique in certain difficult acoustic environments, particularly when the wearer wants to cut out ambient noise but still be able to hear sounds such as speech coming through the headphones. Active hearing protection is also generally better at dealing with low-frequency noise than other types of personal hearing protection. There are disadvantages to this type of device: noise-cancelling headphones are heavier than ordinary earmuffs; they are more expensive than other devices; they require an electrical power source; the electronic circuitry can fail. Sound-cancellation headphones are widely used by aeroplane pilots.

Employees' responsibilities

The onus for hearing protection and the workplace rests not solely with the employer: employees also have responsibilities regarding occupational noise exposure. Employees should wear hearing protection if it is provided and should look after those hearing-protection devices. They should attend any occupational hearing tests that are arranged for them and they should report any noise-related problems they note within their workplace.

Some particular noise challenges

Musicians

Musicians of all genres are at risk of developing noise-induced hearing loss. Many are reluctant to wear ear protection because they feel that it will prevent them hearing the music that they are producing and will therefore impair their performance. There is an element of truth in this, in that the majority of off-the-shelf earplugs allow low-frequency sound through while markedly attenuating high frequencies. This makes music sound dull and lifeless. There are, however, special musicians' earplugs that have a flat frequency response. Three levels of attenuation are available, at 9, 15 and 25 dB. The best way to get these earplugs is to visit a professional audiologist so that an impression can be taken from your ear canal to produce plugs that are moulded to the shape of your ear. The audiologist can also advise which level of attenuation is best for your particular situation.

An even more sophisticated option for musicians is to use in-ear monitoring. In-ear monitors are custom-moulded earplugs with a small built-in receiver (miniature loudspeaker). The earplugs are connected to the sound engineer's mixing desk, either using an electrical cable or wirelessly. The person wearing the plugs is able to adjust the volume to his or her personal requirements. This allows performers to monitor their own performance accurately, at the same time as reducing audience noise and controlling their noise exposure.

Despite all the potential solutions that are available for musicians, many remain reticent about seeking help or even about having a hearing test. They worry that they will be identified as having impaired hearing and no one will then want to employ them. If you are a musician and reading this, we would strongly reassure you that audiologists are bound by the same duties of confidentiality as other healthcare providers and will not divulge the outcome of any tests to a potential employer without your explicit written consent.

Audiences at music concerts are generally less at risk than the performers. However, if you are a regular concertgoer, particularly to concerts with amplified music, it may be sensible to think about investing in a set of musicians' earplugs. People who work in venues where there is amplified music should also think seriously about protecting their hearing.

Motorcyclists

Riding a motorbike is a surprisingly noisy form of transport. This is partly due to the rider's proximity to the engine but more particularly due to noise generated by turbulent airflow past the rider's helmet. Noise reaches potentially dangerous levels at speeds as low as 60 kph (37 mph) and rises to 110 B at 160 kph (100 mph) which, although illegal on public roads in the UK, is regularly exceeded by those motorcyclists who explore their bike's performance on track days at motor racing circuits. Emergency service workers who ride motorbikes are at risk of occupational noise-induced hearing loss, partly because they may need to ride at high speed as part of the job and partly because of the duration of exposure.

The motorcycle press has adopted a very responsible attitude to noise exposure and most motorcyclists in our experience are aware of the potential risk. There are several potential solutions. Fitting a fairing around the front of the bike provides a little extra protection. However, any motorcyclist who is riding regularly or for long distances should wear personal hearing-protection devices. These can be simple foam earplugs or pneumatic muffs that fit within the helmet. Custom-moulded plugs can be produced in a similar way to musicians' earplugs: do-it-yourself kits are available but we recommend visiting an audiologist. In-ear monitors are also available for motorcyclists, and this technology has the advantage of allowing riders to be connected to communication equipment or satellite navigation devices.

Health care

It may surprise many people to discover that healthcare procedures may involve exposure to high levels of sound. Both dentistry and orthopaedic surgery involve the use of powered drills, and in the case of orthopaedic surgery other noisy tools including hammers and powered saws are used. Studies have looked at the amount of noise generated in these situations. Cumulative exposure may reach significant levels for dentists, surgeons or their assistants, but a single exposure is unlikely to reach dangerous levels for a patient. Sound is sometimes used to break up kidney stones using a process called lithotripsy. The noise exposure that a patient receives during this process is unlikely to reach significant levels.

One area where patients are regularly exposed to dangerous sound levels is during magnetic resonance imaging (MRI scanning). In this technique a very high magnetic field has to be generated and switched rapidly on and off. This switching process generates quite high levels of sound. It is very difficult to accurately measure sound levels within a strong magnetic field but estimates suggest that they may reach peaks of 120 dB. MRI scanning departments supply ear protection to wear during the scan and no one should undergo an MRI scan without wearing this hearing protection. Other forms of scanning such as CT scanning are generally quiet and hearing protection is not required.

Excuses that we have heard!

As hearing healthcare professionals it never ceases to amaze us how many people devise excuses as to why they do not need to protect their hearing. We discuss some of the more common excuses below.

I've been clubbing and gigging for years – I get a bit of ringing but it always goes by the following morning.

One problem with noise exposure is that the effects take a long time to appear and are cumulative. This means that for a long time it seems that you are getting away without protecting your ears, but one day you will notice that you aren't hearing as well as other people of the same age. By then the damage has already been done.

I'm a classical musician and classical music doesn't get that loud.

This depends a bit on what sort of classical musician you are. If you are a member of a string quartet, then yes, you can avoid wearing ear protection. If you play in a large orchestra, however, you may be exposed to significant noise levels and ideally you should be wearing some personal hearing protection. And remember, it is not just the performances that contribute towards your noise exposure but also rehearsal times.

I'm a joiner and I use a chop-saw and a router but I'm making quick cuts and therefore I don't need protection.

It is true that a single exposure from one of these tools is unlikely to do harm. But if you are making a 'quick cut' 200 times a day the noise exposure will build up.

> I work on building sites and I have to wear a hard hat, steel toe-capped boots and a high-visibility vest just to get through the front gates in the morning. If I wore all the safety equipment I'm supposed to wear, I wouldn't be able to move, let alone do my job.

Yes, we sympathize with this one. Building sites are among the most dangerous working environments in the UK, and unsurprisingly a lot of safety equipment is recommended. There is no simple answer to this particular problem. We would suggest that you try and wear unobtrusive protection such as foam earplugs. If this is not possible, then at least try and wear hearing protection for the noisiest tasks.

> I work on building sites but I am a plasterer and my job is quiet.

It is not just the noise that you personally produce but also the noise that other people around you make. Your job may be quiet, but if there is a carpenter beside you fixing trim with a nail gun you will be exposed to considerable noise.

> I am self-employed and I simply can't afford hearing protection.

Hearing protection is cheap. We went shopping and had no problem buying a basic but perfectly effective set of earmuffs for about the same as the cost of a supermarket sandwich. For a similar amount of money we were able to buy a dozen pairs of foam earplugs.

> My ears are tough. I don't need protection.

No one's ears are tough. Exposed to loud noise, everyone's ears will eventually show signs of damage.

One word of caution about hearing protection

Although we have stressed in this chapter the importance of looking after your hearing you should only use ear protection when you are somewhere that is genuinely noisy. Your auditory system expects a certain degree of sound input, and if it does not get this input it will increase the central auditory gain. In other words, it will make your hearing excessively sensitive, even to normal sounds. This can lead to the condition called hyperacusis (see page 18).

8

Communication training

One of the most distressing aspects of hearing loss is communication difficulty. Everyday conversation, which was once easy, natural and taken for granted, can start to feel like a real effort. A failed attempt to follow a conversation can leave you feeling frustrated, left out and often exhausted.

Not even the best hearing aids perform as well as fully functioning human ears when it comes to hearing and analysing human speech, especially when listening conditions are difficult. Many people with partial hearing loss find they are still able to follow one-to-one conversation well but have difficulty hearing in a group, at a distance or in a noisy place. There is no perfect solution to these problems and it is still not fully understood how human hearing, when functioning fully, manages to pick out speech in background noise. However, there are a lot of things you can do to make communication easier, less stressful and more satisfying.

Creating a good communication environment

You will probably already have noticed that it's easier to hear in some places than others. It's worth taking some time to think about what factors make a difference. If you find yourself struggling to hear, try to identify all the factors that are making things difficult. If you find you are following a conversation well, ask yourself why that might be. These are the first steps towards creating a good communication environment.

Background noise

Background noise is probably the number one enemy of people with hearing loss! (The exception is people with conductive hearing loss, who tend to get on better in a loud environment.) Much of the time, the amount of noise surrounding us is out of our control and can feel overwhelming. However, we can make wise choices about where we communicate and to some extent we can alter our surroundings to suit ourselves.

At home

Often, within our own homes, we tend to have our conversations while doing something else such as cooking, watching TV or emptying the dishwasher. When someone in the family has a hearing loss, this kind of multi-tasking has to stop. Most people cannot hear well over the clatter of dishes or the whir of a kitchen fan. It's important for everyone in the household to get into the habit of switching off the noise or pausing what they are doing before talking. It may seem like quite an effort at first, but it becomes more automatic with practice. Incidentally, there is some suggestion that constant multi-tasking is not good for our mental health, so other members of the family may benefit from this 'one-thing-at-a-time' approach as well.

At work

It may be less easy to switch off background noise at work, and hearing in an open-plan office or a busy reception area is particularly difficult. However, there are a few steps that might make life a little easier.

- How close are you to noisy printers, photocopiers and air-conditioners? Can you move any further away?
- Is it possible to position your desk in a corner, facing out? That way background noise is at least cut off from two sides.
- When attending a meeting, can you reduce background noise in a room, for example by closing a window or switching off the projector when not in use?

Going out

We can't control the volume of the world outside but we can seek out good communication environments and think about our communication needs when planning ahead. Here are a few suggestions:

- Make a note of local restaurants, pubs and cafes that are communication-friendly. Venues with soft furnishings tend to be easier for hearing than those with a lot of hard surfaces, and small venues may be much easier than larger ones.

- When choosing where to sit, think about background noise. Try to find a place away from the main entrance and away from the clatter of the kitchen. Become adept at spotting audio speakers and avoiding them. If you see a table set for a large group, give it a wide berth – it'll probably get noisy.
- Don't be afraid to ask for music to be turned down. Even people without hearing loss often find it difficult to hear conversation in background noise, so it is likely somebody else will appreciate your request.
- Don't struggle to hear in a car, on a noisy bus or when walking down a main road; it will lead to frustration on both sides. It's far better to postpone the conversation until you get somewhere quieter.

Making the most of visual clues

Everybody uses visual as well as auditory information when communicating with other people. Gestures, facial expressions and body posture give us a lot of information about meaning. To some degree, we all use lip reading to back up what we can hear. Most people aren't aware of lip reading and many of us don't think we can lip read at all. However, if the picture and sound have ever gone out of sync on your digital TV, or if you've ever watched a dubbed film, you'll realize how odd it seems when lip movements and sounds don't match. Here is evidence that our brains are taking lip movements into account when following speech, and we can use this to our advantage.

Although many people find lip-reading classes enjoyable (see the end of this chapter) you don't have to go to a class to be able to use lip reading. Just getting into the habit of watching people's lips when they are talking will make a difference to how much of the conversation you are able to pick up. Of course, you need a clear view of the other person's face, so make sure that you position yourself carefully and that the light is bright enough to see clearly. If you wear glasses, you'll probably hear better if you're wearing them. This may sound odd, but the better you can see the visual clues, the more you will pick up.

Narrowing down the options

It's easier to both hear and lip read when we have some idea what to expect. In lip-reading tests, people do much better when they know the subject beforehand. When going into a new situation, it's a good idea to think beforehand about what's likely to come up; for example, what questions is the doctor likely to ask, or what details are you probably going to be asked for when making an appointment by phone? In some situations, you can narrow down the number of questions you're likely to be asked by being as precise as possible with your request (for example, by stating the time and place you'd like your appointment). A note of caution, though: some people get into the habit of dominating conversations in order to avoid having to work out what other people are saying. This is understandable – talking is less tiring than listening – but unlikely to make you popular!

Getting help from other people

By definition, communication involves at least one other person and therefore you cannot solve all communication difficulties on your own. Even if you've positioned yourself carefully, switched off background noise and put on your glasses, if the person you're talking to has his head in the cupboard or is mumbling you're unlikely to hear what he is saying. Communication requires co-operation.

It may not be enough just to tell people you have a hearing loss. Many people won't know what they can do to help and may do something positively unhelpful, like shouting or over-exaggerating their speech. You will need to give mini-tutorials to people you know and people you meet to tell them how they can help you.

Getting the wording right

It can be hard to make demands of other people. Instructions like: 'You need to slow down and stop hiding your face' can make people feel we are criticizing their way of speaking.

'I' statements tend to come across as less judgemental. 'I have a hearing loss and I lip read. It would help me if I could see your face more clearly and if you could slow down a bit' turns the same ideas into a simple statement of needs.

You might need to spend some time working on how best to explain your hearing needs simply and clearly. You could try out different things and see how people respond. Don't be surprised if you have to explain to the same people again and again; people's minds are full of other things, and they forget.

Chapter 14 of this book deals with how to help someone with a hearing loss, and you might want to give it to your friends and family to read.

Avoiding irritation

As mentioned in Chapter 4, interview studies have often found irritation is frequently mentioned both by people with hearing loss and by their significant others when discussing communication problems. In particular, people tend to get irritated about having to repeat themselves. Sometimes repetition is necessary, but here are a few ideas for cutting down on the irritation it causes.

- Rephrasing a missed sentence can be as effective as repeating it, and sometimes more so. Try asking people to say something in a different way. It might be more helpful for you and less boring for them.
- Sometimes you might have heard part of a sentence but not the whole thing. Try repeating back the part you did hear (e.g. 'What did you say was happening next Thursday?') That way, the other person only has to fill in the gaps, not repeat the whole thing again.
- If you're not sure about part of a sentence, you can check back by saying: 'Did you say . . .?' For example, numbers like 13 and 30 can be hard to tell apart. Instead of saying: 'What was that?', asking: 'Did you say 30?' saves the person from repeating the whole thing again and also stops you from trying to work out which number it was a second time. A 'Did you say . . .?' question prompts a yes or no response.
- Ask people you speak to often to attract your attention before speaking by saying your name or touching your arm. Point out to them that if you are ready and watching from the beginning, they are less likely to have to repeat themselves, so it's worth the effort!

Communication buddies

In a group situation it can be helpful to have a 'communication buddy' nearby who can help you keep up with the conversation. Usually this will be somebody you know well and who you can normally understand quite easily. It's generally much easier to follow a conversation if you know the subject, but sometimes the subject keeps changing and then it's easy to get lost. A communication buddy can help by letting you know what the subject is. Often it will only take one or two words to get you back on track. If it's hard to hear what your buddy is saying amid the other conversation, a couple of words written down on a piece of paper or napkin or typed on a smartphone might do the trick.

Opting out

When you have a hearing loss, communication can be very tiring. Many people find themselves just nodding and smiling, pretending they are still following a conversation they've lost track of. The trouble is, this can lead to embarrassment if somebody suddenly asks you a question or, worse, you smile at a piece of bad news. You will need a break from listening sometimes, but it may be better to explain you're opting out for a while. A trip to the bathroom or a breath of fresh air can be a good pretext for a communication break.

Easier said than done?

Many of the communication tips mentioned above are common sense. It's not difficult to learn what to do, but putting good communication tactics into practice can be more challenging. Changing everyday habits is difficult, and more so when the changes involve asking others to do things differently too.

Having specific goals helps people to make changes and stick to them. So, rather than telling yourself you're going to use better communication strategies, think of a particular situation in which you'd like to communicate more easily (the more specific, the better) then decide exactly what you're going to do in that situation to change things. For example, imagine you always struggle to hear your hairdresser because she talks to you from behind. You might decide: 'When I go for my appointment on Tuesday, I'll explain I have a hearing loss and ask the hairdresser to talk to me face to face first, while we discuss what I want.' It's usually best to start with situations that seem easier, or which aren't so important to you. Once you've had a few successes, you'll gain motivation to change things in more tricky situations.

Formal communication training

While there's a lot you can do in everyday life to improve your communication skills, you may also want to consider a structured training programme.

Auditory training

This form of hearing rehabilitation was first developed after the Second World War, to help soldiers who had lost some of their hearing in battle. It involves listening repeatedly to words and phrases, and the aim is to train the brain to make maximum use of whatever hearing is still functioning. Recent research studies show quite mixed results, but there is some evidence that following an auditory training programme can help people pick out speech better in background noise. It's not entirely clear how auditory training brings changes about, but it certainly doesn't alter anything in the ear. Rather, it's something about the brain's processing of sound which is affected.

These days almost all auditory training programmes are automated and involve doing listening exercises on a computer or a DVD, usually at home. You have to practise very regularly to get any benefit, but only for about half an hour at a time. Auditory training packages are gradually becoming more widespread and are sold by a number of private hearing aid dispensers. Some National Health Service departments can provide them too, although there is normally a charge.

Lip-reading classes

Natural lip-reading ability varies widely between individuals but so far it's not clear what factors make someone a good lip reader – although deaf people are generally better at it than hearing people. Unfortunately, there is a limit to how much people can improve with training, and years of lip-reading tuition does not seem to turn poor lip readers into good ones. Nevertheless, there are several benefits to be gained from attending a lip-reading class:

- You will probably gain more confidence to use lip reading in everyday life.
- You will learn about which sounds are easily confused, which can help you recover from mistakes ('Maybe she said "bin", not "pin"; they look the same').
- You will have a regular opportunity to practise good communication tactics in a supportive environment where mistakes don't matter.
- You will meet other people who also have hearing loss.
- You will probably have fun! Most people really enjoy their lip-reading classes.

Lip-reading classes usually take place at adult education colleges or community centres. Unfortunately there isn't a class in every part of the country. Details of your nearest class can be obtained from the Association of Teachers of Lipreading to Adults (see Resources).

9

Hearing aids and implantable technologies

Hearing aid design and technology is constantly evolving and the developments in this field since the first modern hearing aid was produced in the middle of the twentieth century have been vast. The introduction of digital hearing aids with their inbuilt digital signal processing circuitry has had a major impact, offering improved sound quality and access to many features that contribute not only to better hearing but also to better listening comfort.

The ability to programme and fine-tune a device to someone's unique auditory circumstances and lifestyle needs is one of the advantages of modern hearing instruments today, and a good audiologist will take great care in individualizing the fitting of a hearing aid to match every person's unique situation. The device itself, the setup and fine-tuning will be very different for someone who leads an active, socially participatory life compared to someone who leads a quieter, more sedentary life. This chapter provides an overview of the different styles of hearing instruments that are available today, what patients can expect from fitting and fine-tuning appointments, advice on adapting to your new hearing aids, and a discussion of some of the more commonly asked questions. We also examine the options for those people who are not helped by conventional hearing aids.

Hearing aids have been shown to have a large beneficial impact on quality of life, and with the world's population both increasing and living longer, there are going to be more and more people with hearing loss. It is therefore important from both economic and social aspects to improve provision of hearing health care so that people can remain active participants within their communities.

Analogue versus digital

There is a popular misconception that analogue hearing aids are big bulky devices that fit behind the ear whereas digital aids are tiny discrete aids that fit down inside the ear canal. This is not the case: digital and analogue refer to the electronics inside the aid. Analogue hearing aids, in very simplistic terms, consist of a microphone, an amplifier and a miniature loudspeaker which, rather confusingly, in hearing aid terminology is known as a receiver (see Figure 9.1). Although various filters and gain controls can be built into the amplifier, the device is limited in how much it can process the sound information.

Digital hearing aids also start with a microphone. The information from the microphone is then fed to an analogue-to-digital convertor which, as its name suggests, turns the information into a stream of digital impulses. The now digitized information is sent to a microprocessor, in essence a miniature computer. The microprocessor is programmed with a series of algorithms that enable it to modify the signal. Later in this chapter, we will discuss some of the processing strategies that can be applied. Some of the programmes are built into the microprocessor but others can be manipulated by

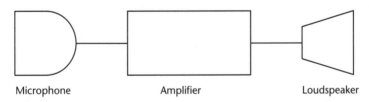

Microphone   Amplifier   Loudspeaker

Figure 9.1   Diagrammatic representation of an analogue hearing aid

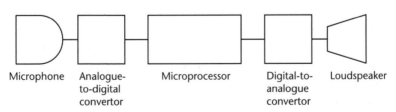

Microphone   Analogue-   Microprocessor   Digital-to-   Loudspeaker
             to-digital   analogue
             convertor   convertor

Figure 9.2   Diagrammatic representation of a digital hearing aid

the audiologist by attaching the hearing aid to an external computer and setting the aid to the person's individual requirements. The signal is then turned back into an analogue signal before going to the miniature loudspeaker (see Figure 9.2, p. 71).

To complicate matters further, there is a type of hearing aid known as a hybrid aid: this combines an analogue aid with some digital control circuitry. The majority of hearing aids supplied by both the NHS and private audiology companies in the UK are now digital.

Hearing aid styles and types

When you first start investigating hearing aids the terminology can seem utterly daunting: there is an avalanche of acronyms describing the different shapes of hearing aid and each manufacturer seems to use different terminology for the features contained within its aids. There are many factors that impact on the kind of device that is recommended for you, such as the pattern and severity of your hearing loss, size and shape of your ear canal, lifestyle and listening demands. Your audiologist will work closely with you to find the best solution that will address both your auditory and lifestyle needs.

When you first start investigating hearing aids the terminology can seem utterly daunting: there is an avalanche of acronyms describing the different shapes of hearing aid and each manufacturer seems to use different jargon for the features contained within its aids. We will try and disentangle this jumble, but before we start we should point out that not every type of hearing aid is suitable for every person. The range of hearing aids that are suitable for you will in part be determined by the pattern and severity of your hearing loss and the size and shape of your ear canal. Your audiologist will be able to advise in this respect.

Behind-the-ear (BTE) hearing aids

BTE hearing aids have the main aid tucked behind the ear (Figure 9.3) and are the most commonly used type of aids in the world. Many people in the UK associate BTE aids with the original analogue NHS hearing aids that their parents or grandparents wore and assume they will be of limited benefit and prone to whistling feedback. This is not the case: today's BTE aids are smaller and less obtrusive and have digital electronics and anti-feedback circuitry. They are extremely adaptable, can be used with almost any ear canal shape and can suit a wide range of hearing losses, from mild to profound. They have a variety of coupling options to the ear, either via a traditional earmould and tubing or via a very thin tube and soft silicone dome that fits in the ear canal.

A selection of much smaller, micro or mini BTEs are now widely available: these generally use a very thin tubing and silicon dome in what is often referred to as an 'open-fit' configuration. Open-fit aids do not block the ear canal in the same way as many other styles of hearing aid and are therefore more comfortable to wear for most people. The first open-fit aids were somewhat prone to feedback and could therefore only be used with relatively minor hearing losses. Improvements in hearing aid circuitry have addressed this feedback issue and such aids are now appropriate for many more people than previously.

Although many people with hearing aids want their aids to be as inconspicuous as possible, there is an initiative not to hide hearing loss, which is traditionally an invisible disability, but to be proud of wearing a hearing aid and even show it off like an accessory. Consequently, many hearing aid companies now also offer their BTE instruments in a range of bright colours and even with interesting graphics and prints on the casing. BTE instruments are easy to handle and are typically more stable and less prone to breakdown compared to in-the-ear devices. BTE aids are

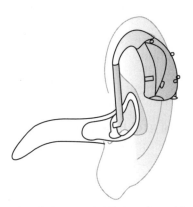

Figure 9.3   A behind-the-ear (BTE) hearing aid

also roomy, in contrast to some other styles, and therefore can have larger controls and can hold more electronics and a larger battery.

In-the-ear (ITE) and in-the-canal (ITC) hearing aids

ITE aids fit in the conchal bowl of the ear – the hollow bit of the outer ear just behind the opening of the ear canal. ITC aids are slightly smaller than ITE aids, sitting over the opening of the ear canal (Figure 9.4). There is nothing behind the ear but they are visible when viewed from the side. They are often selected because they are perceived as being a more cosmetically attractive solution than BTE aids. This is obviously a very personal decision, but in many cases we feel that a thin-tube, micro BTE aid offers a more satisfactory cosmetic and comfort solution. Today there is a wide range of ITE devices available on the market, but they are mostly prescribed in the private sector because of higher associated costs and maintenance and durability issues that make them less attractive for public health organizations. ITEs are more suitable for milder or moderate hearing losses owing to their size.

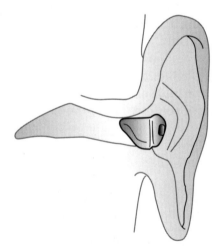

Figure 9.4 An in-the-canal (ITC) hearing aid

Completely-in-the-canal (CIC) and invisible-in-the-canal (IIC) hearing aids

Very often people who are prescribed hearing instruments for the first time will say, 'I want the small, invisible ones that go inside the ear.' Even smaller than ITE aids, CIC and IIC instruments go completely into the ear canal and are invisible to all but the most detailed scrutiny (Figure 9.5). They have a tiny plastic stalk and knob attached so that the wearer can remove the aid when necessary. Because of their size you need to have good manual dexterity for insertion, removal and battery changing. Again, they tend to be best suited for mild to moderate hearing losses and for patients who don't need many advanced features, as there is limited space within the aid for complex electronics.

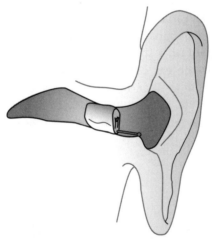

Figure 9.5   An invisible in-the-canal (IIC) hearing aid

Extended-wear hearing aids

An interesting development in hearing aid design is the launch of extended-wear instruments. These are small aids that are designed to be placed very deeply into the ear canal by specially trained clinicians. They are then worn on a semi-permanent basis, being replaced by the clinician every few months. Conventional BTE and ITE hearing aids are taken off during the night, while extended-wear devices are worn for an extended period without taking them off. Extended-wear aids are invisible, allow showering and offer some sonic advantages. They do, however, require regular replacement, and although water resistant they are not completely waterproof. Wearers are advised not to engage in regular swimming or diving.

Receiver-in-the-ear hearing aids (RITE)

As discussed above, the miniature loudspeaker of a hearing aid is called a receiver. The receiver is normally located within the body of the hearing aid. In the case of BTE aids, sound is then conveyed to the ear canal via hollow plastic tubing. In RITE aids the receiver is taken out of the main hearing aid casing and put in the ear canal. A fine wire connects the main body of the aid to the receiver.

Receiver-in-the-canal hearing aids (RIC)

RIC hearing aids are similar to RITE aids but the receiver is inserted deeper into the ear canal (Figure 9.6). These types of hearing aid are sometimes known as canal receiver technology (CRT). The receiver is usually mounted on a soft plastic dome similar to open-fit aids. This means that the ear canal is not occluded, and this style is usually comfortable to wear. Because the microphone and receiver are further apart, RIC aids are less prone to feedback than open-fit aids and hence can be used with more severe hearing losses.

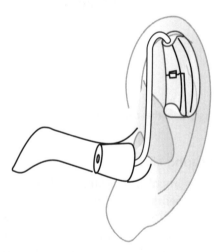

Figure 9.6   A receiver-in-the-canal (RIC) hearing aid

Other styles of hearing aid

Body-worn (BW) aids are rectangular boxes containing batteries and electronic circuitry, connected to an earpiece by a fine electrical cable. The microphone is located in the main box, which is usually clipped to the wearer's clothing. This is not a very cosmetically attractive solution and is rarely prescribed nowadays, but the relatively large size of the device means that these aids can be very powerful.

Various types of hearing aid can be built into the frames of spectacles. This is a solution that is attractive to existing spectacle wearers as wearing BTE hearing aids and spectacles simultaneously may be uncomfortable for some users. Most modern BTE hearing instruments, however, are lighter and smaller than before and it is possible to wear these along with your glasses without their being cumbersome.

Hearing instrument features

Hearing aids have a wide range of features or technologies embedded into their circuitry that all aim to improve your ability to hear speech, provide better listening comfort and give good sound quality.

Directional microphones

The standard hearing aid microphone is omnidirectional. In other words, it picks up sound from all around the wearer. This is useful when you are outdoors or in an environment where you want to be able to hear what is going on from all directions. However, there are many other occasions when you may want to focus on a single sound source and cut out background noise. Listening to someone speak amid the babble of a busy restaurant is a good example of this. A directional microphone is helpful here as it will only pick up sounds from a fairly narrow arc in front of the user. Directional microphones are available on most BTE and some ITE instruments and do improve speech understanding in noisier environments. The user can switch between omnidirectional and directional microphones. Some of the latest hearing aids have sophisticated, automated directionality options that do this switching automatically.

Noise reduction

Digital hearing aids can be programmed to cut out noises as diverse as traffic noise, wind noise or chinking glasses. Such features have been shown to provide more comfort and reduce fatigue from having to concentrate very hard when listening in a noisy situation, but to date have not been shown to improve someone's speech understanding.

Volume controls or remote controls

One thing that surprises people who upgrade from an old analogue hearing aid to a modern digital aid is that often there is no volume control: most modern aids now have automatic volume control built into the microprocessor. There are, however, some hearing aids that do still have volume controls, either on the aid itself or on a separate remote control. If you feel that it is important to have a volume control, this is something that you should discuss with your audiologist.

Wireless technology

As in so many facets of modern life, wireless technology, particularly Bluetooth, is creeping into the world of hearing aids. It is possible to wear two hearing aids that communicate with each other wirelessly. This allows the aids to do what is called binaural processing, improving the audio performance. This technology can be used for other purposes, such as allowing the wearer to make adjustments (e.g. changing the volume control or programme) to one aid, with the other aid being automatically adjusted at the same time. Wireless technology also enables hearing aids to connect to other wireless-equipped devices such as telephones and MP3 players. This is discussed in more detail in Chapter 10.

Telecoil or loop system

The telecoil or loop system is an older but still useful form of wireless technology. This is discussed in Chapter 10.

Feedback manager

One of the most noticeable things about older hearing aids was the fact that they tended to whistle or produce feedback. Modern hearing aids now have much improved methods and technologies of minimizing acoustic feedback but the problem has not been completely eradicated. Your audiologist will be able to programme your hearing aid and run a feedback manager tool to help reduce the likelihood of your hearing aid whistling. A feedback manager is an umbrella term that is used to describe a variety of strategies to help combat feedback, and generally the more sophisticated hearing aids use technologies known as feedback phase cancellation. Other approaches may include techniques called notch filtering or gain reduction.

Extended bandwidth

Hearing aids typically cover a frequency range from 250 Hz to 6,000 Hz. Some devices can amplify at higher frequencies than this and such aids are becoming more widely available. Extending the bandwidth to approximately 10 kHz can bring about improvements in sound localization, speech understanding and generally better sound quality. In most hearing-impaired people the nature of their hearing loss is such that they cannot access very high-pitched sounds.

Frequency-lowering technology

If you have no useful hearing at high frequencies but worthwhile hearing at lower frequencies, it is possible to use algorithms that effectively compress high-pitched sounds down into the hearing range. This technology has been shown to be very effective for children who are still learning language. The jury is still out on how effective this technology is for adult patients, but it may be something that your audiologist will suggest trying.

Data learning and data logging

Many hearing instruments have the ability to perform data learning, which means that the aid will learn your user preferences over time and then automatically apply those changes. If you are consistently turning the volume of your aid down when you are out in a busy street, the hearing aid will learn this and turn itself down once it recognizes that you are in a noisy street situation.

Data logging is a feature that records how and in which environments the hearing aid is being used. The benefit of this is that it helps your hearing healthcare professional to fine-tune the instrument more precisely to your requirements. Data logging can reveal interesting points like forgetting to switch off your aids at night, not using a specific programme, or the fact that you tend to use your hearing aids mostly in noisy environments. Information like this helps the audiologist to act appropriately, for example repeating instructions on how to switch off the hearing aid and save on battery life, removing unwanted programmes or optimizing settings for use in noisy environments.

Tinnitus programmes

Tinnitus is generally most noticeable in quiet surroundings. With many of the hearing aid strategies we have discussed in this chapter, the aim is to make speech clear and remove as much other noise as possible: this is fine when you are having a conversation but can make things too quiet for people with tinnitus at other times. One solution is to have a hearing aid with switchable programmes. You then have a 'listening programme' with all the sound-cancellation features enabled and a 'tinnitus programme' with those features turned off. This means that you get the best of both worlds: when you want to chat, the aid concentrates on making speech clear; when you are pottering around on your own, the sound cancellation circuitry is switched off and the aid will then pick up more ambient environmental sound, giving a useful contrast to the tinnitus.

Another solution is to build a small sound generator into the aid. This can be switched on when you are in quiet surroundings and produces low levels of non-intrusive sound that distracts the brain from the tinnitus. Most hearing aid manufacturers now have aids in their range that incorporate tinnitus sound therapies.

Battery technology

Previous generations of hearing aids relied on mercury batteries, but nowadays less environmentally injurious zinc-air batteries are used. There are also some modern aids that feature rechargeable batteries – these aids are put in a recharging station connected to a mains electricity outlet when not being used. Some recharging stations have other features, such as a programme that dries the aids while they are being recharged or one that checks the electronic circuitry of the aids. Non-rechargeable batteries can represent a significant cost over the lifetime of the aid, so it seems likely that rechargeable technology will become more common. Extended-wear hearing aids (see p. 75) have special batteries that are designed to last for several months.

Implantable devices

Although hearing aids suit a wide variety of hearing losses, there are some exceptions where either the degree of the loss or the medical condition of the person's auditory system requires a different solution. Today there are various implantable technologies that can also be considered for someone with certain types of hearing loss. Your clinician will be able to advise you on whether you are a suitable candidate for this type of treatment. Implantable options include cochlear implants, middle ear implants, bone-anchored hearing aids and auditory brainstem implants.

Cochlear implants

Typically, cochlear implants become an option when someone's hearing loss falls outside the range of what even the most powerful hearing aids can amplify. In other words, they are for people with severe or profound hearing losses who have not benefited from normal acoustic hearing aids. There are very strict candidacy criteria to identify those individuals who are likely to succeed with cochlear implants, and potential patients undergo extensive testing to check whether this solution will be a viable option.

Cochlear implantation involves a major surgical operation to insert a wire electrode into the cochlea. The electrode is connected to a device comprising of electronic circuits, a radio receiver coil and a powerful magnet. This device is embedded underneath the skin in a shallow recess cut in the bone behind the ear. The person wears a device on the outside of the ear that resembles a bulky hearing aid. This device has a radio transmitter coil fitted with another powerful magnet. The external coil is placed over the internal coil and the magnets keep the two coils adjacent to each other. The external device picks up sounds and turns them into radio frequency signals, which are passed via the coils to the internal electronics. These then send electrical impulses to the electrode in the cochlea, which provides direct electrical stimulation of the auditory nerve. This gives sound perception to the brain, but people who have received cochlear implants having gone deaf after previously being able to hear normally report that the perception is very different from normal hearing. The operation to insert the electrode usually destroys whatever residual hearing is present in the operated ear.

Recently surgeons have tried inserting shortened electrodes in an attempt to conserve whatever residual hearing is present. This has been used for people who still have some useful low-frequency hearing but no hearing at higher frequencies. The person then wears an external device that is a combination of a cochlear implant processor and a conventional hearing aid. This is called combined electro-acoustic. In the UK profoundly deaf children are offered bilateral cochlear implants, usually implanted at a single operation. Qualifying adults generally only get a single implant.

Middle ear implants

Middle ear implantation is a relatively new technology and is sometimes recommended for people who are unable to use conventional hearing instruments. Again, stringent criteria apply and candidates are carefully selected only after other avenues have been exhausted. The surgery entails implanting electronics under the skin that are not dissimilar to those used in cochlear implantation. But instead of sending signals to an electrode in the cochlea the electronics are connected to a small mechanical device attached to the ossicles in the middle ear. Information from an external processor is sent to the internal electronics, which make the middle ear device vibrate. This energy is then sent to the cochlea through the normal ossicular chain route.

Bone-anchored hearing aids (BAHA)

It is possible to insert a small titanium screw into a piece of bone under carefully controlled conditions in such a way that the bone cells grow into the material of the screw and the two structures essentially fuse together. This technology was originally developed for dental implants, but it was realized that it would be possible to attach a special type of hearing aid to a screw that had been driven into the bone of the skull above and behind the ear. Sound energy can then pass from the aid, through the screw, into the bone of the skull and directly to the cochlea, bypassing the outer and middle ear entirely. Bone-anchored hearing aids may be used in people with single-sided deafness or certain conductive hearing losses. This includes people with intractable ear infections, absent ear canals, some people with Down's syndrome and some others. The screw passes through the skin and the area must be kept fastidiously clean to prevent infection. The aid is also not very cosmetically attractive unless the person's hair is long enough to cover it. Despite these downsides it is very useful for a group of people who have few other options.

Auditory brainstem implants

Auditory brainstem implants can be a solution for people who have hearing loss because of absent or destroyed auditory nerves, most typically due to a condition called Neurofibromatosis Type II. This is a rare condition and consequently very few of these operations have been performed around the world. The surgery uses the same technique and much of the same equipment as for cochlear implantation, but instead of stimulating an electrode that has been inserted into the cochlea the internal device is connected to an array of electrodes that are placed on the surface of the brainstem.

The fitting appointment(s)

Once you have made the decision to improve your hearing and communication by wearing hearing aids, you will be invited to an appointment with your audiologist. During this appointment your audiologist will use the results from your hearing assessment (audiogram, speech test results, speech-in-noise results, lifestyle and auditory needs analysis) to prescribe a hearing aid that will best fit your profile. If a decision has been made to supply an open-fit or receiver-in-the-canal hearing aid, the audiologist will proceed with fitting the aid. If not, an impression will need to be taken from your ear canal to manufacture the mould for a BTE aid or the body of an ITE aid. This involves first putting a small sponge deep in your ear canal to prevent the impression material going too deep. Then the audiologist mixes two components of a fast-setting putty and squirts the mixture carefully into your ear canal using a blunt-ended plastic syringe. Once the putty has set, which takes a few minutes, the impression and sponge are removed and sent off for manufacture of the appropriate component.

When the aid or mould is ready, the audiologist will see you for a fitting appointment. This usually takes around 1–1.5 hours, and during this time the audiologist will programme your hearing aid(s). Ideally the audiologist should check that the aids are working optimally by using a technique called real ear measurement (REM). This is a short procedure taking approximately 5–10 minutes, and involves putting a fine soft silicon tube attached to a microphone into your ear canal. A loudspeaker in the room produces sounds of known intensity. The sound that reaches your ear canal is measured, first without the hearing aid in position and then with the hearing aid in place and switched on. Based on the results of these measurements your audiologist might make some programming adjustments to the hearing aids. Once the clinician has completed the real ear measurements, the final settings will be programmed into the aid. Your audiologist will then spend the remainder of the appointment discussing the various controls on your hearing aids, cleaning and maintenance, how to change the batteries, where to obtain new ones, and an indication of how long these should typically last. You will also be shown how to insert and remove the hearing aids and the clinician will ask you to practise a few times in the clinic with him or her, just to ensure you are confident in handling the instruments. You will be given some written information to take home, but even so it is often a good idea to bring a friend or relative to the appointment as a lot of information is given and there is a lot to remember.

One of the first things people notice is that their own voice sounds strange or a bit hollow, or echoes. This is a very normal reaction and occurs because of the fact that your ear canal now has something in it that blocks it to some extent. It is important that you give yourself a bit of time to get used to this. If, after two weeks, you are still not used to the sound of your own voice, please go back to your audiologist so he or she can investigate how to help you further.

Getting used to your hearing aids is a process, and it is important that you allow some time to adjust to how it sounds and feels. Some individuals adapt to hearing aids quickly, while others may take a bit longer. On average, most people acclimatize to hearing aids within four weeks, but many people take longer and anything up to 100 days is normal. Once you start to wear your hearing aids it might be best to start off by using them only for an hour a day, in quiet surroundings such as in your home watching television. Gradually build up the time every day, and once you are used to them in the home environment try using them outdoors and in noisier places like shops or restaurants. Building up gradually will ease your brain into listening to many sounds that you may have forgotten about, like birdsong or the hum of the refrigerator, fans or computers. Everyday sounds from crashing cutlery or running water may sound strange at first, but if you allow yourself to gently get used to these then the process of adjusting to life with hearing aids won't be overwhelming.

Some people think that wearing hearing aids causes their hearing to deteriorate further. This is a common misconception and not true at all. Wearing hearing aids provides auditory stimulation to the auditory brain, so hearing aids are actually very good at improving your listening skills. Indeed, the hearing and auditory processing abilities get worse if no amplification is worn, and therefore it can be argued that it is best to start wearing hearing aids sooner rather than later.

The follow-up appointment

Once you have had an opportunity to acclimatize to your hearing aids, you will be invited to attend a follow-up appointment. Depending on how you were getting on with your devices, this appointment can happen anything from two weeks to three months after your first fitting appointment. Some hospital departments and even private practitioners offer a telephone follow-up service. This can be quite convenient and save you a trip coming into the department. If, however, you are struggling to hear over the phone even with your hearing aids, or if the aids need to be adjusted, then a visit to the clinic will be needed. This appointment usually lasts between 30 and 60 minutes.

During the follow-up visit the audiologist will want to check if and how you have worn your hearing aids. He or she will also talk to you about the perceived sound quality, perform listening checks on the aids and make sure that they are comfortable to wear.

Questionnaires will often be used to ascertain how the devices are benefiting you. If any adjustments need to be made to the programming of the hearing aids, the audiologist will connect the devices to the computer and fine-tune them to the desired effect.

A follow-up appointment is a good opportunity to be reminded of various other special features like additional listening programmes and how to use these. The audiologist may reiterate advice on care and maintenance of the aids, including battery changing and replacement services. He or she might refer you to lip-reading classes, recommend additional auditory training programmes, suggest the use of assistive listening devices and provide general counselling. In addition, you will be given information on what to do if your hearing aids break down or you lose them.

Looking after hearing aids

Caring for a hearing aid depends on the individual aid and you should be given specific instructions – both written and verbal – from your audiologist. There are some general principles, however. The electronics in hearing aids need to be kept dry, so do not use water to clean the main part of the aid: gentle rubbing with a soft cloth or tissue is enough. The plastic of most hearing aids can be damaged by many cleaning solvents so these should be avoided. If you have a BTE hearing aid, the main aid can be separated from the mould and tubing. The mould and tubing can then be washed in soapy water, remembering not to reconnect them to the main body of the aid until they are completely dry. Some aids are supplied with little brushes to remove wax and dirt: use these as shown by your audiologist. Do not poke the brushes or other implements into openings in the main body of the aid unless your audiologist has told you that it is safe to do so. There are proprietary devices for drying hearing aids: some are containers filled with desiccant materials; others are electrically powered and use gentle heat. Some electrically powered dryers also feature ultraviolet light which helps to kill micro-organisms on the aid. As always, check with your audiologist about what is best for your particular aid.

Troubleshooting

From time to time your hearing aids may stop working properly. It is useful to consult the hearing aid instruction manual that was provided when you first obtained them, as it may contain helpful ideas that will help you problem-solve on your own. If you are unable to do this, then it is best to make an appointment with your audiologist. Some of the common problems that can easily be resolved are listed in Table 9.1.

Table 9.1   Some common problems affecting hearing aids

Problem	Cause	Solution
Hearing aid is weak or dead	Battery run down	Replace battery
	Sound outlet is blocked	Clean sound outlet/ change wax filter
	Microphone opening is blocked	Clean microphone opening with brush
	Volume control is down	Turn up the volume control
Hearing aid is intermittent or distorted	Aid switched to telecoil	Switch aid to microphone mode
	Corroded battery	Replace battery
Hearing aid squeals or whistles	Aid not inserted properly	Remove and re-insert aid
	Ear wax blocking ear canal or tubing	See GP for wax removal or clean tubing

One ear or two?

There is substantial evidence that shows it is better to listen with two ears rather than with one, and we would suggest having aids for both ears. In fact, the benefits of binaural hearing are such that if cost is a factor it is usually better to opt for two cheaper hearing aids rather than a single expensive aid. The benefits of wearing two hearing instruments include:

- better overall sound quality;
- better ability to understand speech, particularly in a noisy environment;

- greatly improved ability to locate sources and direction of sound;
- a sense of balanced hearing;
- more relaxed hearing.

However, we are pragmatists and understand that, for a variety of reasons, many people will opt for just a single aid. One aid is certainly better than no aid. If you do opt for a solitary aid, we suggest you allow yourself time to get used to it and then ask yourself if it is doing everything you hoped or whether you would be better getting another aid for the other side. If you reach the latter conclusion, have a chat with your audiologist. If you are opting for a unilateral hearing aid and the hearing in your ears is different, you can make an argument for fitting the aid to either the better-hearing ear or the worse-hearing ear: have a chat with your audiologist about the pros and cons.

When two hearing aids have been prescribed, they are generally colour-coded: a small red mark for the right ear and a blue one for the left.

Can I get my hearing aids over the internet?

From time to time there are newspaper and internet advertisements that try to lure individuals to purchase hearing aids through the post or via the internet. We do not recommend this type of service delivery. Obviously, as hearing healthcare professionals we are biased, but we really feel that everyone with a hearing problem should be assessed by an appropriately trained professional. This allows the cause of your hearing problem to be ascertained, important underlying conditions detected and a range of solutions discussed. Inappropriately fitted hearing aids may not only fail to supply benefit but can even damage the hearing. Buying an aid over the internet also means that hearing-impaired people miss out on the significant after-care that can only be provided by a face-to-face meeting with a trained professional.

What are the pros and cons of private and NHS aids?

It used to be the case that the NHS only provided analogue hearing aids, so many people who wanted a digital aid went to a private hearing aid supplier. This is no longer the case, as almost all NHS aids are now digital and in some cases are exactly the same aids as those supplied by private hearing aid companies. The big advantage of NHS hearing aids is that you do not have to pay for them: the NHS essentially gives them to you on long-term loan. If you lose one and need a replacement, there is sometimes a charge, but otherwise the service is included in standard NHS provision. This applies not only to the aids but also to batteries.

There are several reasons why people choose to go to a private hearing aid supplier. It is often easier to obtain an appointment at a time that suits you. The service is usually quicker – both the initial consultation and the turnaround time for the manufacture of the aid. Private hearing aid suppliers are more likely to have the latest state-of-the-art devices and more likely to have a large range of aids to offer you. NHS clinics generally do not offer ITE aids except in special circumstances: if you want to investigate this style you should contact a private supplier.

Private hearing aid suppliers are also generally more flexible regarding follow-up visits. Some people find that they need their hearing aid regularly reprogrammed: this can be difficult to arrange in some NHS services. If you buy a private hearing aid, the manufacturer generally gives a worldwide two-year warranty. Private hearing aid suppliers will often sell their hearing aids as part of a package that includes servicing costs and batteries for a variable length of time, and some of these deals also include extended warranties. If you do opt for a private hearing aid, you should ensure that it is included on your general household insurance policy.

Provision of NHS aids is changing and many private hearing aid suppliers now also fit NHS aids. The range of aids that they can fit under their NHS contract is limited and does not generally include ITE aids.

I've heard a new aid is coming out. Should I wait?

The pace of hearing aid development is so rapid that there will always be a new aid just around the corner. Most developments are small incremental changes rather than dramatic redesign. We therefore recommend that once you have made your mind up to try a hearing aid, you should try one of the available options rather than holding out in hope of something better.

Single-sided deafness and hearing aids

In this chapter we have made the tacit assumption that most people seeking hearing aids have hearing loss in both ears. This is generally the case, but there are some people who have normal or near-normal hearing in one ear and a significant or complete loss in the other. If the affected ear still has some hearing, it is possible to try a conventional hearing aid. However, if the loss is greater than this a hearing aid may not be able to help. It is possible to use various technological solutions to try and rehabilitate this loss. CROS aids are one option. CROS stands for contralateral routing of signal, and essentially it means that the signal on the side of the deaf ear is re-routed to the normal hearing side. This enables sound information from the deaf side of the body to be fed into the hearing ear. CROS systems used to link the two parts with a wire running around the back of the wearer's head, but many people found it very difficult to get on with this design. Wireless CROS systems have recently entered the market and are proving much more satisfactory. With a CROS setup the sound delivered to the good ear is not amplified. BiCROS is an acronym for binaural contralateral routing of signal, and such systems are used when someone has a hearing loss in one ear and no hearing in the other ear. With a BiCROS setup the sound information from the side with no hearing is sent to the good side. On the good side the device amplifies the sounds from both sides of the body using conventional hearing aid technology.

Bone-anchored hearing aids can be used in a similar fashion to CROS aids for single-sided deafness. The bone-anchored hearing aid is attached to the deaf side of the head. It then transmits sound energy into the bone of the skull. This is conducted through the bone to the normal cochlea on the other side of the head. There has been some experimental work looking at whether cochlear implants have a role in the management of single-sided deafness, and some encouraging initial research suggests that cochlear implants may be helpful in ameliorating severe tinnitus if that is present on the deaf side.

10

Hearing assistance technology and language service professionals

As discussed in earlier chapters, hearing aids are not equally helpful in every situation. Moreover, there are times when you won't be wearing your hearing aids (such as in bed or in the bath) when you still need to be aware of sounds around you, particularly things like doorbells or smoke alarms. Fortunately, a great deal of extra technology is available to help. The term 'hearing assistance technology' (HAT) is sometimes used to mean any technology other than hearing aids and it can broadly be divided into two categories: assistive listening devices and alerting devices. It includes things which are very straightforward, such as a louder telephone bell, and quite complex devices which enable you to connect your hearing aids up to your smartphone or computer.

Unfortunately, research shows that awareness of hearing assistance technology is very low, among both hearing aid users and audiology professionals in most countries. This chapter aims to outline what kind of technology is available and how you can obtain it, so you have the information to ask for what you need. It also gives some information about professionals who can help in situations that demand a high level of listening.

Linking up to assistive listening devices (ALD)

If you have a hearing aid, there are several ways in which you can link up to an assistive listening device. All of them enable sound from a remote microphone to be transmitted directly into your hearing aid. Normally, if you are listening to a sound far away from you, it becomes weaker as it covers the distance between you, and by the time it reaches your hearing aid microphone it is less intense than when it started. ALDs eliminate the effect of distance and give you the impression that the sound is coming right into your hearing aid(s) from nearby. Another advantage is that background noise can be cut out. When you connect to an ALD you normally disable the ordinary hearing aid microphone, so you don't hear all the other sounds around you but only what is coming through the remote microphone. Some hearing aids allow you to connect to an ALD while keeping the hearing aid microphone switched on at the same time. This is useful if you need to listen out for something, for example the doorbell.

Telecoil

Most BTE hearing aids and many ITE ones have a telecoil fitted inside as standard. Cochlear implant receivers have them too. This enables the aid to pick up signals from a loop system wherever one is installed and switched on. The 'loop' refers to a wire which needs to completely surround or be very close to the hearing aids in order to create a magnetic field which can be picked up by the telecoil. It can be small enough to wear around your neck or large enough to cover a whole auditorium. Many telephone receivers have loop systems built into them, and you can get special neck loops to plug into mobile phones. Once an audiologist has activated the telecoil, you switch the hearing aid to the T position on the aid itself or on the remote control when you want to use this facility. Not all hearing aids have this function, and even if they do it is not always enabled within the device. So, if you are envisaging needing this technology, discuss it with your audiologist and ensure that he or she has turned on the telecoil within the aid.

Direct audio input

For some behind-the-ear hearing aids and cochlear implant receivers, you can get an extra piece (sometimes called a 'shoe') that clips on to the end of the aid and allows you to plug a special wire into it. The other end of the wire can be connected to a radio aid, FM system or other personal listening device (see p. 94). You can also use it to connect your hearing aid(s) directly to an MP3 player, radio or computer.

Bluetooth

In recent years, it has become possible to use some hearing aids with Bluetooth technology, although not all hearing aids are compatible yet. In addition to your hearing aids, you need a special 'Bluetooth streamer', which is a small device worn around the neck. Once you have this, you can connect wirelessly to up to eight different electronic devices such as a personal listener, mobile phone, computer, MP3 player or TV. Bluetooth works with a digital radio signal so interference shouldn't be a problem.

Hearing assistance technology in public places

Larger loops are common in public places like banks, post offices, theatres, places of worship and lecture theatres. Premises with loop systems are typically identified with a sign featuring a diagram of an ear with a T in the bottom right corner (see Figure 10.1). Wherever you see a sign like this, you should just be able to switch your telecoil on and make use of the loop. It can be particularly helpful at a counter where there is a glass panel between you and the person serving you; switching on the loop is like taking the panel away. It can also help in places where you might otherwise

Figure 10.1   The sign in public buildings indicating that a loop system is available for use with the telecoil or T setting in some hearing aids

be bothered by noises around you. You will hear less rustling from your popcorn-eating neighbours in the cinema and less background chatter at a busy reception desk. You do need to ensure that you are inside the loop, and even then you will find that there are areas of good reception and poorer areas within it. There is a degree of trial and error in finding the best position.

Unfortunately, many people report trying to use a loop system or similar only to find that it's switched off or not working. If this happens to you, make sure you point it out to staff. If enough people mention it, it's more likely that something will be done. If you are going to a performance, it's a good idea to mention beforehand that you'll be using the loop, as sometimes it only covers certain seats.

Some theatres and cinemas use an infrared system instead of a loop. This involves having an extra little box, normally worn round the neck, to pick up the infrared signal. You will need to request one of these at the box office. You still need to switch on your telecoil to use it, but an advantage of this system is that people who don't have hearing aids can still use the amplifier with a pair of headphones. There is usually no charge for borrowing this equipment although you may have to leave a deposit.

If plays or stage shows are difficult for you to follow even with a loop system, quite a lot of theatres now put on captioned performances. One or two of the shows in a run will have surtitles displayed on a screen above the stage, so you really will follow all the dialogue. Some cinemas put on subtitled versions of films too, and of course foreign-language films have the advantage of always being subtitled.

If you need to use the phone when you're out, all of BT's public payphones in the UK have a telecoil installed and most have amplifiers. Some also have a textphone available (see p. 98).

Personal listening device

This is a versatile portable device which can be used with headphones or with a hearing aid (using the telecoil and a miniature loop or direct audio inputs). The headphones, loop or direct audio cable connect to a small, hand-held box which has a microphone and volume and tone controls. Whatever sound is received by the microphone is then fed to the headphones or hearing aid. This is useful for situations such as being a passenger in a car: the microphone is clipped to the driver's clothing, enabling you to hear him or her above the engine noise. These devices can also connect to equipment such as televisions. Basic devices link to the TV via a wire but more sophisticated devices can operate using wireless technology, which means you continue to hear the sound even if you move to another room. Personal amplifiers can also be used in conjunction with a Bluetooth streamer.

Equipment for use at home

There are many types of equipment you can use at home to make your life easier, more convenient and safer. In the UK, some equipment is available free of charge through social services. Provision varies a great deal across the country, as does waiting time, but it is certainly worth contacting your local social services to see what they can provide before buying anything. The sensory impairment team normally deal with equipment and they will probably arrange some kind of assessment of your needs.

Special smoke alarms for deaf and hard of hearing people can be provided by the UK Fire Service. These have flashing lights and a vibrating pad you can put under your pillow to wake you up. If you contact your local fire brigade, they can organize a free fire safety assessment of your home at which they can offer general advice, as well as arrange for a smoke alarm to be fitted.

British Telecom customers who have a hearing loss are entitled to a free 'tone caller' which amplifies the ringer of your telephone and can be placed anywhere in your home.

Equipment is available to buy from some hearing aid dispensers and from a number of specialist suppliers. You can order equipment online or by sending off an order form from a catalogue.

Home entertainment

A wide range of equipment is available to help you hear the television and radio better. The same equipment can normally be used for various kinds of music players (CD, MP3, etc.) and computers. Personal amplifiers can be used in this situation but there are many other potential solutions.

Domestic loop system

This is a small version of the loop system you find in churches and cinemas. It needs to be installed in your living room. A box of electronics is connected to your TV or other audiovisual equipment – most loop systems have a range of inputs such as microphone, line or SCART connections. The sound signal from the TV is then sent from the loop device through a thin wire that is normally fixed to the skirting board. Once it is installed and switched on, you only need to switch on the telecoil in your hearing aid to be able to use it from anywhere in the room. The volume and tone can be adjusted by the loop device and other people will still be able to hear sound coming out of the TV speakers at their chosen volume.

Infrared amplifier

This device has two parts: a small infrared box placed close to your TV or radio and a headset or neck loop with infrared receiver, which you wear. There are no wires and the sound is clear, but it will not work if anything comes between the two parts or if you wander about.

Plug-in headphones

For music in particular, many people prefer to take their hearing aids out and listen through a set of good-quality headphones. This normally means the sound is only heard by you.

Which equipment you choose depends very much on your needs, your budget and your lifestyle. A few questions to consider are:

- Do you normally watch or listen on your own, or do other people need to hear the sound at the same time at 'normal' volume?
- Are wires across the room going to cause a problem with small children, pets or people unsteady on their feet?
- Do you normally watch or listen in one spot, or do you like to be able to move around?
- Do you already have hearing aids and are they fitted with telecoils?
- Do you prefer to keep your hearing aids in or take them out?
- Do you often watch or listen away from home?
- Are you able to use small controls, or do you need something quite 'chunky' and easy to adjust?

Subtitles

Depending on the degree of your hearing loss, you may find TV easier to follow with subtitles. Even if you hear well with a TV amplifier most of the time, subtitles can be helpful for certain programmes with a lot of background music, or when people speak with unfamiliar accents. Subtitles are accessible via all digital TV providers and you can normally switch them on simply by pressing the subtitle or 'SUB' button on your remote control, though increasingly TV manufacturers use a graphical representation on the remote – check with your TV's manual. You can also select subtitles when you use a TV catch-up service via your computer.

Most commercial DVDs enable you to switch on subtitles via the menu. Note that 'English (hard of hearing)' subtitles describe important sounds such as 'phone ringing' while 'English' subtitles only show the dialogue. On some internet sites, the term 'captions' is used for subtitles in the same language as the spoken words (while 'subtitles' means in a different language). Not all DVD recorders record subtitles but there are models which can. Most PVR systems can also be set up to record subtitles.

Telephones

Landlines

Many ordinary home telephones have a telecoil built into the receiver, and it's worth checking yours. If it doesn't, you will just hear a buzz when you switch your hearing aid to telecoil. If you wear a behind-the-ear hearing aid, you will also hear better if you hold the receiver a little higher than normal, so the sound enters your hearing aid rather than hitting the earmould inside your ear.

If the phone is unclear in spite of trying these steps, there are a number of options to choose from.

Adapting your existing telephone

You can buy either a portable amplifier that straps on to the telephone earpiece or a plug-in amplifier that goes between your phone and the receiver cord. These are both inexpensive options, but they won't fit all models of telephone.

Buying a new phone

There are many phones available with built-in amplifiers. Some boost the volume just a little, while others are very powerful. Most will reset when the call is finished to avoid the sound being dangerously loud for people with normal hearing. Both fixed and cordless models are available, and some have extra features like large buttons or a second receiver, allowing another person to listen and assist with the conversation. Most also allow you to choose the pitch and volume of the ringer. If you have a conductive hearing loss, you may hear better with a special receiver that you press against the bone behind your ear instead of the ear itself.

Textphones

Sometimes known as Minicoms, textphones have a keyboard and screen and enable you to communicate in writing over the phone line. You can communicate directly with another textphone, or via an operator, with a person using a conventional phone. While many public services still have a textphone number, they are becoming less widespread with the increase of text communication via mobile phone and instant messaging or emailing via computer.

Mobile phones

A lot of people get interference if they hold a mobile phone up to their hearing aid. Various types of neck loop and direct input lead are available to attach to your mobile phone, or you can use a Bluetooth streamer. All these devices cut interference and make the sound clearer. Some people find that just plugging in a standard headset and listening with this (instead of a hearing aid) makes the phone clear enough. Not all devices are compatible with all makes of phone, so check the details before you buy. Virtually all mobile phones can be set to vibrate so you don't need to worry about missing the ringer.

Alerting devices

A common problem for many people with hearing loss is missing sounds like the doorbell and alarm clock. This can make a big difference to how comfortable and secure you feel when on your own. Fortunately several solutions are available, some of which are quite simple.

Stand-alone devices

The least costly devices deal with just one piece of equipment at a time. You can get telephone ringers and doorbells that ring extra loudly and/or activate a flashing light. You can also get alarm clocks (as well as smoke alarms) with vibrating pads which you place under your pillow to wake you up. Baby monitors with flashing lights and vibrating pads are also available.

Pager systems

If you need several alerting devices, it can be more convenient to use a pager system. You can place transmitters next to your doorbell, your phone, your baby monitor, your cooker, etc., and a receiver clipped to your clothes will vibrate when any one of them is activated. A small light will indicate which device has gone off. Most pagers come with additional vibrating pads for use at night time. They are generally more expensive than stand-alone systems, although people with more severe hearing loss can sometimes obtain them from local social services.

Wired-in systems

It may be possible to have an alerting system wired up to your house lights, so that the lights flash on and off when the phone or doorbell rings. This is usually done via social services, but has become less common with the availability of more sophisticated pagers.

Hearing dogs

Hardly a 'device', but an alternative method of being alerted to sounds around the home, hearing dogs are specially trained to respond to sounds like door bells and alarms by finding and touching their owners, rather than barking. They lead you to the source of the sound or lie down quickly for a danger signal. Hearing dogs are normally allowed in public places, like guide dogs, and their owners often report that they feel more confident with their dog by their side. The dogs – which can be any breed – are trained and pro-vided by a charity, Hearing Dogs for Deaf People, and there is quite a rigorous assessment if you want to apply for one. Usually they are only provided to people with severe or profound hearing loss.

Equipment and services for work and education

If you are working, your employer is required under the Equality Act (see Chapter 11) to provide any additional equipment or service that you may need in order to do your job effectively. This may include things like a loop system, a different telephone or a speech-to-text reporter (see p. 101).

The 'Access to Work' scheme can help with funding (see Chapter 11) but, ultimately, equipment provision is your employer's responsibility.

If you are in higher education, you can apply for a Disabled Student Allowance, which you can spend either on equipment or services like note-taking, or on a combination of both. The amount you get depends on the severity of your hearing loss and the hours per week you are studying.

If you are taking a course for your own interest, rather than for a formal qualification, you should still have access to equipment to help you hear the instructor better. Most adult education centres have a disability officer who should be able to tell you what is available.

Listening devices

Most of the listening equipment available for home use can also be used in a classroom or meeting room. However, there are a few special considerations:

- A domestic loop is probably not adequate. Commercial loops are available for larger areas and should be fitted as standard in modern classrooms, lecture theatres and conference halls. However, many older buildings do not have them.
- In places without a room loop you can use a personal listening device (see p. 94). You will probably hear single talkers well if they speak through a microphone attached to their clothes or on a podium which links to your device. However, a wireless system will probably be much more practical than a hard-wired one.
- In many classes and meetings you will sometimes need to listen to more than one person talking. The further away the talker is from the microphone, the worse the sound quality. For optimal hearing, a microphone needs to be passed from one talker to another. Where this is not practical, long-range microphones

can be used and placed in the middle of the table or hung from the ceiling. You can get directional table-top microphones which you can swivel yourself to face the person who is talking. Some are much better quality than others, but there is always the problem that a microphone far from the talker will pick up background noise to some degree.

If you work at a counter with a loop system for the public, this can be adapted so that you – on the staff side – are able to benefit from it too. The same is true of loop systems in taxis.

Telephones

If you need an amplified telephone at work, you will need to check whether the model you want is compatible with the phone system. If it isn't, there is usually a way around the problem which your telecommunications department should be able to sort out. Incidentally, don't be afraid to request an amplified phone even if you share a phone with several people. Many workers with normal hearing like to be able to increase the volume for a caller with a quiet voice or when the surroundings are noisy.

Alerting devices

Your employer is responsible for the safety of all employees. If you are unable to hear audible alarms, a flashing light or personal pager should be provided for you.

Language service professionals (LSP)

This is the name for a group of specially trained people who provide support services for deaf and hard of hearing people. They include the following:

- Note-takers take notes in classes or lectures on behalf of a student who cannot take his or her own notes because of the need to keep looking up to lip read. Normally this is done on a laptop, but notes may be written by hand.
- Speed typists rapidly type a summary of what is being said in a lecture or meeting as it is being said. The deaf person reads from the laptop screen. Alternatively, a larger screen is used for several people.

- Palantypists transcribe what is being said word for word. They use a special keyboard which enables much faster typing than a conventional one.

Collectively, all of the above are known as speech-to-text reporters. Normally the typist will sit next to the deaf person, but sometimes the service is provided remotely via Skype.

Other language service professionals include:

- lip speakers, who say whatever the speaker is saying but without voice; they are trained in clear speech and sometimes fingerspell difficult words;
- sign language interpreters, who translate what is said into sign language. Specialist sign interpreters exist for deaf–blind people.

Note-takers are often students studying other courses and they can normally be booked via the university or college's disability office. Other LSPs normally need to be booked through an agency. Several agencies exist and it is worth bearing in mind that travel expenses are normally charged as well as fees, so it will usually be cheaper to opt for a local organization. It is also important to book as far in advance as possible, as most kinds of LSP are in short supply.

If you are attending a hospital appointment (in the UK), it should be possible to request an LSP directly through the hospital's Patient Advice and Liaison Service (PALS) rather than having to approach an agency yourself.

Other considerations

As awareness of both HAT and LSPs is low, you will probably have to be quite proactive in obtaining the additional equipment or services you need. Don't be afraid to take an equipment catalogue along to your employer or institution (or to show them a web page) as they are quite unlikely to know already what's available. You may need to do a fair bit of research yourself.

Some private companies offer a money-back guarantee on equipment, and this is useful if you're not quite sure what would be most helpful. In some parts of the UK there are drop-in sessions, operated either by the NHS audiology department or social services, where you can try out some types of equipment, but this is still fairly uncommon. You may need to go through a bit of trial and error before you end up with the equipment that is right for you, sending equipment back to companies or social services and exchanging it for something different. If your NHS audiology department has a hearing therapist, he or she should be able to offer appropriate advice.

As well as persistence, a fair degree of assertiveness is needed when you start to use HAT. You might have to complain at a counter where the loop is not switched on or to ask a guest speaker to wear a microphone for you. Most personal listeners are more visible than hearing aids and it will be obvious to other people at a meeting that you are using a speed typist. For this reason, you need to be comfortable wearing hearing aids out and about and telling people about your hearing loss before you start using many types of extra technology. Once you have done some work on this (see Chapter 12) you are more likely to get full benefit from the wealth of additional help available.

Remember that every request or demand you make helps to raise awareness and will make things that little bit easier for other people with hearing loss in future.

11

Your rights

Does hearing loss count as a disability?

Whether or not you consider yourself to be disabled is partly a case of personal identity. Some people do not think that their hearing loss is significant enough to be thought of as a disability, and some people who have grown up using sign language see Deafness as a cultural identity rather than a disability (see Chapter 1). Others feel that using the term 'disability' helps to reflect the seriousness and permanence of their condition. The British government defines disability as 'a physical or mental impairment which has a substantial and long-term adverse effect on your ability to carry out normal day-to-day activities'. Any hearing loss which is significant enough to cause difficulty with everyday communication would probably fit this definition. Being classed as 'disabled' means you are protected and supported by legislation which is outlined in this chapter. However, whether you describe yourself as 'disabled' in your day-to-day life is very much a personal choice.

Registering as deaf or hard of hearing

There is no requirement to register yourself as deaf or hard of hearing, and doing so (or choosing not to) does not affect your rights. However, if most people did register, this would give local government a more accurate idea of how many people with hearing loss live in the area. This should help to influence the planning of local services so that the needs of people with hearing loss are taken into account. In the UK, you can register by filling in a short form available from your local social services.

Equality

Different countries have different kinds of legislation to protect the rights of minority groups. In the United Kingdom (not Northern Ireland) the Equality Act was introduced in 2010. It brings together anti-discrimination laws for all kinds of minority groups, including disabled people.

The Equality Act applies to both work and public services. It makes it illegal to discriminate against disabled people directly (for example, by refusing to serve a deaf customer) and indirectly (for example, by offering only telephone interviews to people applying for a job). The Act also requires employers and services to make 'reasonable adjustments' to meet the needs of disabled people. Such adjustments include things like adapting buildings and providing equipment (such as an amplified telephone or loop system) but also altering the way things are done, for example not requiring a secretary with hearing loss to take minutes at meetings.

Financial help

If you are working and need extra support because of your hearing loss, it is your employer's responsibility to provide it. However, financial help is available in the UK through a scheme called Access to Work. This can help meet the costs of special equipment (such as a loop system) and also support services, such as a speech-to-text reporter at meetings. The scheme can also provide funding for support at a job interview. You can contact an Access to Work adviser through your local Jobcentre Plus.

You may also be eligible for government benefits because of your hearing loss, even if you have a job. The benefits system is undergoing substantial changes at the time of writing and the charity Action on Hearing Loss has a lot of helpful information about this (see Resources for contact details).

Complaining

Just because there are laws against discrimination, this does not mean that it no longer happens. However, you do not have to put up with it! There are many ways in which you can assert your rights, from taking an employer to court right down to writing a short letter of complaint when you feel you have been treated unfairly. Some of the charities for people with hearing loss run campaigns for greater awareness and fairer treatment, so you don't have to be a lone voice. The number of people with hearing loss is steadily increasing and companies cannot afford to lose your support.

Seeking compensation for hearing loss

The following is a brief overview of the compensation system in the UK. It does not apply in other countries and is not a substitute for expert legal advice.

To fulfil the legal requirements for compensation it must be possible to demonstrate three things:

1 There has been exposure to excessive noise levels.
2 There has been a hearing loss as a consequence of that exposure.
3 There was a foreseeable risk of injury from the exposure and appropriate remedial measures were not instituted.

The regulations regarding excessive noise have changed over the years. The current regulations are discussed in Chapter 7, but depending when your noise exposure happened, different criteria may apply. There is also a time period during which a claim should be launched. Generally this is within three years of the excessive noise exposure but courts do have some leeway regarding this.

The first step in pursuing a compensation claim is to obtain appropriate legal representation. If you are a member of a trade union, they may be able to help in this respect. If you do not have trade union support and are arranging this yourself, remember that not all legal representatives are equally experienced in noise-induced hearing loss work. It is worth asking about their relevant experience and doing some shopping around.

Once you have engaged the services of a legal team they will generally arrange to obtain a report from an independent doctor, who in turn will arrange hearing tests. This independent doctor will not be one of your usual ENT or audiology team, though their medical notes will be photocopied and made available to your legal team. There is a complicated set of tables that shows what hearing loss is expected at any particular age and this is subtracted from the results of your hearing test to find what percentage of hearing loss is caused by noise exposure. This figure is then used to apportion compensation.

If your hearing loss was caused by military service, compensation can be sought through the Armed Forces Compensation Scheme or War Pensions Scheme (which scheme applies depends on when you served in the armed forces). Details of these schemes with regard to hearing loss are available from Action on Hearing Loss or the Royal British Legion or, if you are from Scotland, the Royal British Legion in Scotland. Details are in the resources section.

12

Adjusting and coping

Coping with change

Most people like to feel a sense of control over their own lives and hearing loss can take that sense away, at least for a time. If you have developed a hearing loss suddenly, you may well feel as though your whole world has been turned upside down and nothing is as it used to be. Even with a milder hearing loss, you may feel as though changes have been thrust upon you, and this can be hard to cope with. Activities that you used to enjoy, such as socializing with other people, can start to feel overwhelming. You may feel resentful that poor hearing is interfering with the way you want to live your life. You will probably need plenty of time to adjust to life with a hearing loss and you may well experience ups and downs, feeling that you are coping well one day and that it's all too much the next. This is all quite normal. There is no standard amount of time that it takes to adjust to hearing loss and it is not always true that a mild hearing loss will be easier to accept than a more severe one. There are many factors at play, such as your lifestyle, your personality and the amount of social support around you.

Avoiding social withdrawal

While it's important to allow yourself time and space to adjust to your hearing loss, it's also important to try and keep going with your everyday activities as much as you can. People with hearing loss can find themselves withdrawing more and more from social situations. This is understandable: if communication is tiring and frustrating and you feel embarrassed about making mistakes, it's easier just to stay at home.

The problem is that this can quickly develop into a downward spiral. You avoid meeting up with people, and this way you avoid potential embarrassment but you also miss any opportunities for positive conversation, so your fear of embarrassment remains or even increases. Next time you're obliged to socialize with people you are likely to feel more anxious because you're not used to it. Anxiety makes it harder to listen, so there's actually a greater likelihood that you'll make mistakes. Furthermore, spending more time at home on your own gives you more opportunity to dwell on your hearing loss and how bad it makes you feel, and the more you avoid social interaction the harder it becomes to get out and about again.

You probably will have to change some of your activities because of your hearing loss, but you will be able to adapt many of them instead of abandoning them altogether. Can you invite people round instead of meeting at a noisy restaurant? Can you go to a captioned performance at the theatre? Can you use a personal listening device at your evening class? A combination of hearing aids, additional equipment and good communication tactics (see Chapters 9, 10 and 8 respectively) can help to keep you connected to the social world.

Denial and disclosure

It is very common for people to go through a period of denial when they first develop a hearing loss, and this can go on for years. You may tell yourself that people just don't speak as clearly as they used to, or that the sound on your TV has become less distinct, or that the world is just noisier. Even if you are aware yourself that your hearing is not what it used to be, you may be unwilling to admit it to other people. For older people this is often due to the fact that hearing loss is so strongly associated with ageing. Most of us feel younger in ourselves than we actually are and do not want to be labelled as an 'old person'. Research has shown that this is one of the barriers to using hearing aids; people sometimes see them as a sign of old age and want to resist that image, especially in a youth-centred society. Interestingly, younger people don't seem to share that association at all.

Although it can feel like a difficult task, telling other people about your hearing loss can ultimately make life easier. You will need emotional support from the people closest to you and support with communication from just about everyone you meet. You cannot use good communication tactics without co-operation from the person you are speaking to (more about this in Chapter 8) and asking for co-operation normally involves first explaining that you have a hearing loss. Furthermore, *not* disclosing hearing loss can lead to all kinds of negative assumptions on the part of other people. If you apparently ignore someone who greets you on the street, she's likely to think you're rude, and if you give an inappropriate answer to a question she's likely to think you're stupid or crazy, unless you've explained that you have a hearing loss. Most people would rather be known to be deaf than thought of as stupid or antisocial. Some interesting research has also shown that hearing people responded more favourably to a hearing aid wearer who explained he was deaf than to another who never mentioned it.

Broaching the subject of hearing loss is not always easy. Many people fear a negative reaction: that someone will make a joke about it or be stand-offish. Some people worry about an over-sympathetic 'poor you' reaction or that they will be asked lots of questions about their deafness that they don't want to answer. It would be nice to say that none of these reactions will happen, but sadly that is not the case. Some people will react in a way that you do not want them to, and if you have had a bad reaction in the past this can really put you off telling other people. However, the opposite is also true: if you tell somebody about your hearing loss and their reaction is kind and helpful, this will motivate you to tell more people.

To some degree you can control other people's responses by the words and tone of voice you use yourself. Being matter-of-fact and to the point can discourage excessive sympathy, and moving straight on to how to communicate can discourage personal questions. You might want to rehearse different statements and see which feels most comfortable to you (there is more about this in Chapter 8). You could ask a person you trust for his or her opinion.

If you haven't told many people about your hearing loss and you feel quite nervous about it, it might help to make a disclosure plan. Think about all the various people you communicate with in different situations and what difficulties you have with them. Then consider how difficult or easy it would be to tell each person, and why. A typical list is shown in Table 12.1.

You can then decide who to start with. You may choose a person you know quite well and who you think is likely to be supportive

Table 12.1   People you might have to inform about your hearing loss

Person	Importance	Difficulty
Boss	High (I'm making mistakes)	Difficult (he's always in a rush and usually brusque)
Julie at work	Medium (she might have noticed I don't always respond first time)	Quite easy (she's very friendly and chatty)
Hairdresser	Medium (I sometimes don't get what she's asking)	Medium (I don't know her very well and I'm not sure what she'll say)
Doctor's receptionist	High (last time I totally missed my turn)	Quite easy (everyone is there for a medical problem so she won't be surprised)
Woman in café	Low (it's easy to guess what she's saying)	Easy (she has a hearing aid herself)

or you may want to start with someone you only encounter briefly (like a receptionist), just for the practice. Take note of the person's reaction and whether things became any easier afterwards. Once you have gained some experience in disclosing hearing loss, you will probably feel better able to approach people you are more nervous about. If you do get a negative reaction from someone, try not to let it put you off, but ask yourself: what does it say about that person? It's likely that on balance you will get more helpful reactions than unhelpful ones.

Telling people about your hearing loss once does not necessarily mean they will remember. You will need to tell people again if they slip back into poor communication behaviour. This is frustrating, but at least indicates that hearing loss is not the most memorable thing about you.

Taking action: deciding for yourself

Telling people is one of several forms of action you may choose to take in order to help you cope with your hearing loss. Others are starting to use hearing aids, or getting additional equipment, or adopting new communication tactics. You may not feel able to take all these steps at once, and it's important for you to feel ready in yourself.

Research in the field of health psychology shows that people who make their own decisions about what action to take and when are more likely to stick with them than people who are told what to do. Two psychologists, James Prochaska and Carlo DiClementi, suggested that making a change in our lives involves passing through several stages: precontemplation (not even considering it), contemplation, preparation, action and maintenance. They argue that we cannot be forced from one stage into another, but that with appropriate information and support we can be motivated to move through the stages ourselves.

Some people are pressured into getting hearing aids by family members before they feel ready and then end up not using them. If you really don't feel ready to take any action to deal with your hearing loss at the moment (and there can be many reasons for this), simply make yourself aware of what help is available and give yourself time to mull it over. If you are unsure about whether to do something or not (in other words, in the 'contemplation' stage), it can help to weigh up the pros and cons. One tool for doing this is a cost–benefit chart, a template for which is shown in Table 12.2.

Table 12.2   A blank cost–benefit chart

What's good about things as they are?	*What's bad about things as they are?*
What might be better if I made a change?	*What might be bad if I made a change?*

Table 12.3   A cost–benefit chart for someone with hearing loss

What's good about not having a hearing aid?	What's bad about not having a hearing aid?
I can keep hearing loss hidden. I feel 'normal'.	I often mishear in groups. My partner complains the TV is too loud. I don't enjoy the theatre any more.
What might be better if I got a hearing aid?	What might be bad if I got a hearing aid?
I might hear speech better. I could use one of those gadgets at the theatre to hear better.	People would notice. I'd look older. I'd have a new gadget to get used to.

If someone considering whether to get hearing aids were to fill in one of these charts, it might look like Table 12.3.

Writing things down like this can help you to think more clearly and move towards a decision. It can turn a vague feeling of uncertainty into a reasoned argument. You may realize that most of your hesitation is due to a particular barrier which you can overcome, perhaps by getting more information or asking a question at your audiology department. Alternatively, you may decide that the 'cons' outweigh the 'pros' at the moment. If this is the case, put your chart away and look at it again in a few months' time. Has anything changed?

Maintenance

It is one thing to make a change in your life and quite another to stick to it. Many people start wearing hearing aids but then give up. Others start trying to use better communication tactics but then slip back into old habits. There can be many reasons for this. It may be that hearing aids don't meet your expectations or just seem too fiddly to manage. It may be that you feel fed up with continually asking people to face you and speak clearly, only to hear them drop their voice again at the next sentence. It may be that you have other things going on in your life and that dealing with hearing problems is no longer a priority. If you're not getting much support from people around you, it can also be hard to persevere.

It would be unrealistic to expect yourself to work equally hard at coping with your hearing loss all the time. However, it's also unrealistic to think that going through a rough patch means that all your efforts up until now have been wasted. People slide back and forth through the stages of change and you may go through the process of weighing things up and deciding you are going to take action several times over. However, after a time you will probably find that you are in more of a routine, that wearing hearing aids feels more natural and that good communication tactics have become a habit.

Getting support

Coping with any difficult change in life – including hearing loss – is made easier if you feel supported by other people. If you can, it's a good idea to take a partner, family member or close friend along with you when you attend audiology appointments and to involve him or her in your rehabilitation. Everybody close to you needs to adjust to your hearing loss as well as you, so talk about it together. Chapter 14 discusses specific things that people around you can do to help you with communication.

Even with support, hearing loss can feel quite isolating if nobody else in your family or social circle has the same problem. Making contact with others who also have hearing loss can be immensely helpful. This can be done in several ways. If you are lucky, there may be a local support group in your area you can go along to; these are often held in community centres. You may also have a lip-reading class nearby; most of these take place in adult education colleges. It may also be that your audiology department runs group sessions of some kind. Being surrounded by others who are 'in the same boat' can be very encouraging, and people often comment that they enjoy being in a place where communication mistakes really don't matter because everyone is making them. There are some larger national events, such as conferences for people with hearing loss, that you may also like to get involved in.

There are a growing number of support networks running on social media sites such as Facebook, and a number of charities run internet forums where you can ask questions and 'chat' online to other people with hearing loss.

Becoming a member of a national charity such as Action on Hearing Loss (AoHL; see Resources) can also be a good way of feeling connected to the wider world of hearing loss. Receiving a quarterly magazine will help to keep you informed of important developments in research and legislation and will also remind you that you are not alone with hearing loss.

13

The future

We saw in Chapter 6 that there are some types of conductive hearing loss that will either resolve spontaneously or can be corrected surgically. Most people in the United Kingdom with hearing loss, however, do not have one of these conductive losses – their hearing loss is a sensorineural loss due to damage to the inner ear structures or auditory nerve fibres. Most other groups of animals, including amphibians, reptiles, fish and birds, can repair both the hearing and balance parts of their inner ears if they become damaged, but humans, in common with other mammals, have largely lost this ability: there is very limited power of regeneration for the structures involved with balance and almost no facility at all for regeneration of the hearing structures within the cochlea. Thus any damage to auditory structures within the inner ear is usually permanent. The current management of this type of hearing loss is therefore directed towards support and rehabilitation rather than trying to cure the underlying pathological process, and this is frustrating for doctors and patients alike.

Our understanding of the ear has improved greatly: we understand the anatomy of the inner ear and we understand how it functions; we understand how the auditory system develops during the foetal period and we even understand much of how the body's genetic information controls this development. However, being able to use all that information to repair damaged ears is still tantalizingly beyond our grasp.

Although it is often thought that sensorineural hearing loss is caused by damage to the hair cells, this is an oversimplification and there are various different components that can be affected: in addition to the inner and outer hair cells, their associated nerve cells can be damaged or die, and the membranous structures inside the cochlea can deteriorate with time, as can the specialized cells that supply the inner ear with nourishment and maintain the complex chemical balance of the cochlear fluids. Different treatment strategies are needed depending on which element is responsible for the hearing loss, and as yet we have no way of discovering the faulty component without causing further damage to the ear. If we could accurately diagnose which part of the structure was causing the problem, the next decision would be to establish which technique to use for trying to repair the damage. Various methods have been suggested and some have already been tried in experimental models.

One therapeutic option includes the use of drugs to stimulate the cochlea to produce its own new cells. During foetal development a 'brake' is applied to cell division in the inner ear – this is what stops the mammalian ear from repairing itself. Some drugs have been identified that can release this brake, and there is a possibility of being able to introduce such drugs into the cochlea relatively easily via a structure called the round window membrane. This is a thin membrane that separates the fluid-filled space of the inner ear from the air-filled space of the middle ear (Chapter 2). If certain small molecules are injected through the eardrum into the middle ear, they can diffuse through the round window membrane into the inner ear fluids. Using drugs in this fashion to try and improve hearing has been tried in mice and did result in some improvement, though this improvement was very small.

We are all used to hearing news reports about scientific progress in the field of gene therapy, and the use of stem cells and such techniques have been considered with regard to hearing loss. One possible avenue would be to try and introduce genes into cells within a damaged cochlea to make existing non-specialized 'support' cells transform into the missing specialized cells. Alternatively, the genes could make support cells divide to produce new specialized cells. Genes that can do this are already known, one example being a gene called Atoh 1. There has been an experiment where introducing this gene caused regeneration of hair cells in rodents. Other ideas include the use of stem cells – these are cells that have not yet differentiated to form specialized cells and retain the ability to become any cell in the body if they are manipulated correctly. Stem cells can be obtained from embryonic tissue but also from some adult tissue. There have been attempts to grow ear structures from stem cells in tissue culture, outside the body, for later introduction into the cochlea. Alternatively, stem cells could be introduced into a damaged ear and then produce the new structures in situ.

Not only is it difficult to use genes and stem cells to produce new tissue but there is also a risk that having turned one of these processes on, there might be no way of stopping it after enough new specialized cells had been produced to correct the damage. Uncontrolled cell production could potentially result in tumour formation. A further obstacle to using genes or stem cells is how to get these agents into the cochlea. Surgery has been suggested, but this is invasive and risks causing further damage to an already damaged organ. Viruses can be used to get genetic material into cells: a harmless virus or a pathogenic virus that has been treated to make it harmless can have the useful gene added to its genetic material. The virus can then get into the target cell and insert the beneficial gene. This is an extremely complicated process but one that is attracting considerable scientific interest.

Other issues with gene, stem cell and drug treatments for deafness include the time frame for administration: most of the animal experiments have involved causing the deafness and then almost immediately applying the treatment. Most people with hearing loss, by contrast, seek help years or even decades after the damage started to become apparent. We do not yet know whether techniques being used in animals will be transferable to humans. A further issue is that all the techniques discussed above are aimed at regenerating damaged anatomical structures. Producing new cells is only part of the problem: the cells have to function as well as simply exist.

This discussion of gene therapy and stem cell treatments sounds very exciting but these techniques are very much at the experimental stage and there are no immediate plans to start trials on humans.

One area where we may see some development is in the field of cochlear implantation. Cochlear implants are very useful in the treatment of people who have lost all or very nearly all of their hearing. The device that is surgically implanted in the ear provides electrical stimulation of nerve fibres in the cochlea, giving the patient back some degree of sound awareness (for a full explanation see Chapter 9). For this technique to work, there need to be a reasonable number of functioning nerve cells remaining in the cochlea. This is not always the case and is thought to be one reason why cochlear implantation does not work well for every patient. Scientists have discovered chemicals produced by the body that they call neurotropic factors. Experimental work on animals has shown that such factors could increase the number of functioning nerve cells within a damaged cochlea and potentially could improve cochlear implantation outcomes. The neurotropic factors could either be introduced with the implant or the ear could be persuaded to produce its own by use of gene therapy. Although this is an interesting area of research it is probably only ever going to apply to a very small number of people.

Another interesting area that is being explored is trying to prevent – or at least limit – the damage caused by noise exposure. We saw in Chapter 7 how use of earplugs or earmuffs reduces the amount of sound reaching the inner ear and protects against noise-induced hearing loss. However, not all dangerously loud sounds are predictable and it is not always practical to wear ear defenders. One example of this is soldiers, who are generally quite good about wearing ear protection when training, but in real battle they often do not wear their ear defenders as they need to be aware of their surroundings and colleagues.

When the ear is exposed to dangerously loud noises the cells in the cochlea that ultimately die do not do so immediately. Instead, they are labelled by the body as 'cells that need to die' and a complex process called apoptosis is started. This process removes the cell as neatly as possible, recycling much of the useful material contained within the cell. Apoptosis can be triggered by high levels of free radicals and is controlled by a complicated biochemical pathway that uses several enzymes, particularly a group of enzymes called caspases. This gap between the exposure to dangerous sound and the ultimate death of the cell lasts for hours or possibly even a day or two and hence offers a potential therapeutic target: if the apoptosis could be blocked, the cell might survive.

Various trials are underway to work out how this could be achieved. One avenue being explored is to use antioxidants to try and mop up free radicals before they can start the apoptosis process. Two drug trials are being conducted: one uses a combination of vitamins A, C and E together with magnesium, known as ACE Mg. The other uses an amino acid called d-methionine, often abbreviated to D-met. The idea is that if people are given one of these treatments prior to sound exposure, any free radicals that are produced will be neutralized before they can set off the cascade that eventually destroys the cochlear cell. There is also the even more exciting possibility that these treatments could be given immediately after sound exposure and still be effective. A related area being investigated is whether the enzymes used by the apoptosis process could be blocked. To date no suitable drugs for this have been identified.

Free radicals may also be implicated in the cochlear damage that can follow the use of certain anti-cancer drugs or powerful antibiotics, and it is hoped that the treatments that are being investigated for noise damage to the cochlea may also be effective for patients receiving one of these ototoxic drugs.

We hope this short chapter has given you some insight into the type of research that is being carried out to try and overcome hearing loss. It also demonstrates the complexities that are confronting researchers. We hope that this research will eventually provide better solutions for people with hearing loss, but we think that such solutions are still quite a long way from fruition.

14

When someone you know has a hearing loss

This chapter is written for the benefit of people with good hearing who regularly spend time with a person with hearing loss. It might be your partner, a relative, a friend, a colleague or somebody you look after. You may find it helpful to read other parts of this book too, particularly the sections on the psychosocial effects of hearing loss (Chapters 4 and 12).

Frustration is normal!

Trying to communicate with someone who has a hearing loss can be very frustrating. In particular, having to keep stopping and repeating what you have just said can really take the pleasure out of conversation. Even when you know that it isn't the other person's fault, you can end up feeling irritated, and it can be particularly upsetting when the two of you used to be able to chat easily. These feelings are only human.

However, while conversation with a hearing-impaired person is rarely as easy as between two people with normal hearing, there are things you can do to reduce frustration on both sides. This chapter will give you a few ideas.

Things to keep in mind

Before looking at specific things you can do to help, here are a few general points to be aware of.

Hearing aids are not the whole solution

Sometimes family members believe that if they can only persuade their loved one to get a hearing aid, everything will be all right. Sadly, this is not the case. Hearing aids are not like glasses, which (for most people) restore vision to normal. Although most people do find hearing aids helpful, listening with them is not the same as having perfect hearing. There are some situations – especially noisy ones – in which they do not help very much. If the person you know with hearing loss has or is getting hearing aids, you will still need to learn about other ways of helping.

Communication involves vision as well as hearing

All of us use visual clues (body language, facial expression) to help our understanding of what is being said, but this is particularly important for people with hearing loss. Some people rely very heavily on lip reading to follow conversation, while others deny any lip-reading ability at all. Nevertheless, visual clues are crucial to people with hearing loss, even if they are not always consciously aware of using them.

Sometimes it's easier to hear than other times

A common complaint from people who live with a hearing-impaired person is: 'He hears when he wants to.' Having to repeat one question five times while getting an instant response to another can make you feel that the person simply is not making enough effort to listen. The truth is that some environments are much more difficult for hearing than others (something simple like switching on a noisy kettle can make all the difference) and some words are much easier to hear than others, depending on what speech sounds they contain and what type of hearing loss the person has. Moreover, listening with a hearing loss is tiring, and it might not be possible to sustain concentration for as long as a hearing person can. Of course, people with hearing loss are as capable of ignoring an unwelcome request as anyone else, but it might not always be a case of deliberately tuning out.

Making communication easier

Here are a few suggestions for things to do – and avoid – when talking to someone with a hearing loss, to increase your chances of being understood.

Do

- Do make yourself visible. Probably the single most helpful thing you can do is make sure your whole face can be seen clearly so that the person can lip read and see your facial expression. This may involve getting up and shifting position, switching the light on, breaking off from what you were doing or changing lifelong habits such as covering your mouth when talking. It will also involve reminding yourself to stop talking every time you need to look down or turn away.
- Do slow down. Fast speech makes words merge together and so is harder to follow. However, don't slow down so much that your speech loses its natural rhythm.
- Do speak clearly. Some people have naturally clear speech, while others don't. It can be hard to change your way of speaking, but it isn't impossible. Thinking about articulating the beginnings and ends of words can be a good start.
- Do reduce background noise. The person with hearing loss will probably hear you better if there isn't other noise going on at the same time. Switch off or move away from the noise whenever you can before you start a conversation.
- Do give a signal that you are going to speak. A person with hearing loss who is focused on something else may not realize you are talking to her until you are part way through, by which time she cannot catch up. Saying the person's name, then pausing, or touching her arm, will alert her to listen.
- Do try saying it a different way. Rephrasing can sometimes be more helpful than simply repeating, probably because some words are easier to hear and lip read than others. It's also less tedious for you.

Don't

- Don't shout. If someone cannot hear, we naturally make ourselves louder, but this is rarely helpful. Hearing aids do a pretty good job of making things louder; it is the clarity of speech that people with hearing aids lack. Shouting actually makes speech less clear and can even sound painfully loud through hearing aids. Furthermore, it makes whatever you are saying seem aggressive, even if this is far from your intention.

- Don't over-exaggerate. Clear speech is helpful, but exaggerated mouth movements make everything look distorted and are harder to follow.
- Don't say: 'It doesn't matter!' The remark you are making may seem trivial to you and not worth repeating, but to a person who has been working hard to hear it, it's important.

Getting into new habits

A lot of the advice above involves changing the way you do things. People who see a lot of each other get into all sorts of comfortable communication habits, such as talking from different rooms in the house or chatting with the TV on. Getting out of old habits and into new ones is hard and doesn't happen overnight. You need to keep on practising and not be too hard on yourself if you sometimes forget. With enough practice and patience, good communication can become as habitual as anything else.

Going to hearing appointments

Some more individualized communication advice might be available from your local audiology service. Almost all audiology departments invite 'significant others' to attend appointments. As communication affects both of you, it makes sense for both of you to go along and discuss your communication needs and priorities. If hearing aids are being fitted, it is also helpful for you to learn how to put them on and maintain them. They can be hard to get used to and two minds are better at retaining information than one.

Giving communication support

If you are close to a person with hearing loss, you may well find yourself needing to support him or her in situations which involve a lot of communication with other people, such as going to doctor's appointments or meeting up with friends and family. It's hard to see the person you're with struggling to cope, and you may find yourself using 'rescue behaviour', such as jumping in to answer a question he or she didn't hear, or having a conversation with a health professional on his or her behalf. People usually do this kind of thing to protect their loved one from awkwardness and embarrassment, but in the longer term it can make the person with hearing loss feel weak, dependent and lacking in self-confidence.

It is better to speak up for the person with hearing loss and let other people know what they can do to help. You can share your own experience in a friendly way ('I'm finding it really helps to slow down a bit'). Sometimes you might need to be quite assertive about refusing to answer on your loved one's behalf. Some people deliberately step or look away to make sure remarks have to be addressed to the person with hearing loss.

This is not to say that you have to leave the hearing-impaired person to sink or swim! You can give support by, for example, letting him know what subject is being discussed in a group, or asking him a clear question which will get him back into the conversation if he is getting lost. Writing down a name or a couple of words can be enough to get somebody back on track if the topic changes, so it's useful to keep a pen and paper handy (or just type on your smartphone!).

Lifestyle changes

As well as offering communication support, you can help with social situations by planning them with hearing in mind. If, for example, you are arranging a family gathering, think about the venue. If you are meeting up in somebody's house, can a quieter seating area be set up where the person with hearing loss can talk to different family members one at a time? If you are going to a restaurant, can you choose somewhere small, without lots of background music? Can you invite people to tea in two small groups rather than one large one? Might a catch-up on a country walk be easier than a catch-up in a noisy pub? Social life is important to nearly everybody, but all too often people with hearing loss find themselves dropping out because communication is too hard. You have an important role to play in helping the person with hearing loss find alternative ways of keeping socially connected.

Having said this, do not lose sight of your own needs! One of your roles in life may now be a supporter of a person with hearing loss, but it is not your only role. People who live with a hearing-impaired person often find they miss out on social events such as parties and theatre trips, even though their own hearing is unaf-fected. If you are missing events you used to enjoy, perhaps you can join up with friends once in a while. People who are fulfilled in their own lives are generally more effective in supporting others who are facing difficulties in theirs.

Resources

General self-help, information and support

UK

Action on Hearing Loss (formerly **Royal National Institute for Deaf People**)
19–23 Featherstone Street
London EC1Y 8SL
Tel.: 0808 808 0123; textphone 0808 808 9000 (both freephone)
Website: www.actiononhearingloss.org.uk

National Deaf Children's Society
Ground Floor South, Castle House
37–45 Paul Street
London EC2A 4LS
Tel.: 020 7490 8656
Freephone helpline: 0808 800 8880 (9.30 a.m. to 9.30 p.m., Monday to Thursday; 9.30 a.m. to 5 p.m., Friday)
Minicom: 020 7490 8656
Website: www.ndcs.org.uk

The website also gives details of offices in Belfast, Birmingham, Cardiff and Glasgow.

Overseas

Australia

Better Hearing Australia
Better Hearing House
5 High Street
Prahran, Victoria 3181
Tel.: 1300 242 842 or (03) 9510 1577
TTY: (03) 9510 3499
Website: www.betterhearingaustralia.org.au

The website gives details of offices in all other Australian states.

Canada

Canadian Hard of Hearing Association
2415 Holly Lane, Suite 205
Ottawa, Ontario K1V 7P2
Tel.: 613-526-1504
TTY: 613-526-4718
Website: www.chha.ca

Ireland

DeafHear.ie
35 North Frederick Street
Dublin 1
Tel.: 01 8175700
Minicom: 01 8175777
Fax/Text: 01 8783629
Website: www.deafhear.ie

USA

Hearing Loss Association of America
7910 Woodmont Avenue, Suite 1200
Bethesda, MD 20814
Tel.: 301 657 2248
Website: www.hearingloss.org

Hearing Health Foundation
363 Seventh Avenue, 10th Floor
New York, NY 10001
Tel.: 212 257 6140
Website: www.hearinghealthfoundation.org

Support for UK service personnel

Royal British Legion
199 Borough High Street
London SE1 1AA
Tel.: 020 3207 2100
Freephone: 0808 802 8080
Website: www.britishlegion.org.uk

The Royal British Legion Scotland
New Haig House
Logie Green Road
Edinburgh EH7 4HR
Tel.: 0131 550 1583
Website: www.rblscotland.com

Support for specific conditions and associated symptoms

UK

British Acoustic Neuroma Association (BANA)
Tapton Park Innovation Centre
Brimington Road, Tapton
Chesterfield
Derbyshire S41 0TZ
Tel.: 01623 632 143 (general); 0800 652 3143 (freephone)
Website: www.bana-uk.com

British Tinnitus Association
Ground Floor, Unit 5
Acorn Business Park
Woodseats Close
Sheffield S8 0TB
Tel.: 0114 250 9933 (general); 0800 018 0527 (freephone)
Minicom: 0114 258 5694
Website: www.tinnitus.org.uk

The Ménière's Society
The Rookery
Surrey Hills Business Park
Sheephouse Lane
Dorking
Surrey RH5 6QT
Tel.: 01306 876 883 (general); 0845 120 2975 (helpline)
Website: www.menieres.org.uk

USA

Hyperacusis Network
4417 Anapaula Lane
Green Bay, WI 54311
Website: www.hyperacusis.net

Miscellaneous

Association of Teachers of Lipreading to Adults (ATLA)
Website: www.lipreading.org.uk

My Baby's Hearing
Website: www.babyhearing.org/index.asp

NHS Newborn Hearing Screening Programme
Website: hearing.screening.nhs.uk

Noise at Work (UK)
Health and Safety Executive
Website: www.hse.gov.uk/noise/index.htm

Further reading

Hearing

Alpiner, J. and McCarthy, P., *Rehabilitative Audiology: Children and adults.* Lippincott Williams and Wilkins, Philadelphia, 2000.
A professional text written in an accessible style.

Coleman, N., *The Train in the Night: A story of music and loss.* Jonathan Cape, London, 2012.
A personal account of hearing loss and learning to cope, especially with regard to the author's main passion, music.

Graham, J. and Baguley, D. (eds), *Ballantynes's Deafness.* Seventh edn. Wiley-Blackwell, Oxford, 2009.
Intended for healthcare professionals but written in a very accessible format.

Lodge, D., *Deaf Sentence.* Penguin, Harmondsworth, 2009.
A novel from one of the world's great writers who has a hearing loss himself. It gives great insight into hearing loss.

Tait, V., *Life After Hearing Loss: Telling it like it is.* Hearing Link, Eastbourne, 2007.
A collection of interviews with people affected by hearing loss.Several other excellent autobiographies of Deaf, deafened and hard of hearing people are also available in bookshops.

Tinnitus

Baguley, D., Andersson, G., McFerran, D. and McKenna, L., *Tinnitus: A multidisciplinary approach.* Second edn. Wiley-Blackwell, Oxford, 2013.
Intended for healthcare professionals but covers all the current theories and approaches.

McKenna, L., Baguley, D. and McFerran, D., *Living with Tinnitus and Hyperacusis.* Sheldon Press, London, 2010.
A companion volume to this book. There is some inevitable overlap but tinnitus and hyperacusis are covered in much greater detail than in this volume.

Tyler, R. (ed.), *The Consumer Handbook on Tinnitus.* Auricle Ink Publishers, Sedona, Arizona, 2008.
A collection of chapters written by leading tinnitus specialists and covering a range of subjects.

Index